PORTABLE *Reiki*

Easy Self-Treatments for Home, Work and on the Go

TANMAYA HONERVOGT
with Carol Neiman

D1370500

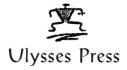

Ulysses Press

Published in the U.S. in 2006 by
Ulysses Press
P.O. Box 3440
Berkeley, CA 94703
www.ulyssespress.com

First published as A GAIA BUSY PERSON'S GUIDE TO REIKI in the United Kingdom in 2005 by Gaia Books Ltd, an imprint of Octopus Publishing Group

Library of Congress Control Number 2005908286
ISBN 1-56975-529-9

Editor	Jonathan Hilton
Editorial Direction	Jo Godfrey Wood
Interior Design	Peggy Sadler
Cover Design	Robles & Zubeldia
Art Direction	Patrick Nugent
Production	Louise Hall
Photography	Ruth Jenkinson
Proofreading and Index	Kathie Gill
U.S. Proofreader	Amy Hough

Printed and bound in China

10 9 8 7 6 5 4 3 2 1

Distributed by Publishers Group West

Contents

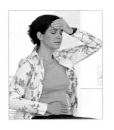
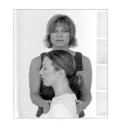
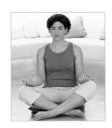
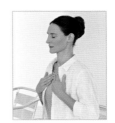

Introduction

"The word *healing* comes from the same root as the word *whole*. Whole, health, healing, holy … all come from the same root. To be healed means to be joined with the whole. To be ill means to be disconnected with the whole. An ill person is one who has simply developed blocks between himself and the whole, so something is disconnected. The function of the healer is to reconnect it. But when I say the function of the healer is to reconnect it, I don't mean that the healer has to do something. The healer is just a vehicle; the doer is the whole."

Osho, *From Medication to Meditation*

Intuitively, most of us understand that real "health" is much more than just the absence of disease. When we are functioning at our optimum best, we have a sense that the body, mind, and emotions are all working together in harmony. Not only do we feel good physically, we also experience clarity, vitality, and a vibrant joy in being alive.

In the fast-paced world of today, we face many obstacles in maintaining this quality of true health. We have too much to do, and too little time in which to do it. Our efforts to tend to our own needs are often thwarted by the demands of the workplace. Our attempts to establish the comforting routines and rituals that help us to relax and reflect can be disrupted by unexpected crises or sudden shifts in our priorities. Some studies show that more than 60 percent of those who seek medical attention are suffering from stress-related illnesses.

As the medical profession has begun to recognize that so many of our modern illnesses are rooted in stress, researchers have started to take a fresh look at Eastern methods of healing and meditation. Clearly, there are limitations to a mechanical approach to health, one that treats just the symptoms of these diseases without addressing their causes. The East has a long history of exploring the deep interdependency of body, mind, and spirit. And many Western medical professionals now recognize the value of Eastern techniques in developing a more holistic approach to supporting health and well-being.

This book introduces the basic techniques and principles of one such Eastern technique, Reiki, as a natural way for the reader to support his or her own health and well-being in daily life. The Reiki treatments in this book will be beneficial even without formal training and initiation. If, after experimenting for a few weeks and experiencing the benefits that flow from it, you feel drawn to exploring it more deeply, you might want to participate in a seminar to receive training and an "attunement." These seminars and attunements are given by certified Reiki Master-Teachers, and greatly enhance the power and effectiveness of Reiki techniques.

THE ORIGINS OF REIKI

Reiki (pronounced "ray-key") is a method of healing that has its roots in ancient Tibetan practices that were used to harmonize and heal the body, mind, and spirit. The word *Reiki* is derived from the Japanese, and means "universal life energy." The syllable *rei* describes the boundless, cosmic aspect of this energy; *ki* is the vital life energy itself.

Reiki is a natural conduit or channel for this universal life energy. Its fascinating history has been passed down from teacher to student since the nineteenth century, when a Japanese monk named Dr. Mikao Usui rediscovered the principles of Reiki after a long search. Dr. Usui's search began in a quest to understand the healing miracles of Jesus, and ended in a deeply personal and profound healing transformation. After this experience, Dr. Usui devoted the remainder of his life to healing others and passing on the teachings of Reiki. The Usui System of Natural Healing, named after Dr. Usui, has now spread throughout the world and has helped many people to live healthier, more relaxed, and more vibrant lives.

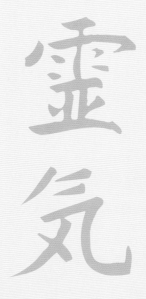

BASIC REIKI PRINCIPLES

Reiki works with the endocrine system and regulates hormone balance in the body and metabolism. On an energetic level, the endocrine glands correspond to and interrelate with the "chakras" in the energy body.

In ancient Eastern wisdom, there are seven main chakras. Each of these chakras is a vital energy center in the body that serves to receive, transmute, and organize the subtle energies of the cosmic life force. This life force, or *ki*, is manifested in the human organism and is called *chi* in Chinese or *prana* in Sanskrit, which is the ancient language of India. In Western terminology, we sometimes refer to it as "light" – and it is present in all living things, including plants and animals.

This powerful natural energy is available to all of us. We are born with it, and it flows through us and sustains our lives every day. It is this energy that we draw on in the course of our daily activities. And if our lives were perfectly in balance, it would be naturally replenished through our interactions with others in a loving environment, and with rest and relaxation, fresh air, clean water, and wholesome, natural food. Of course, our lives are not perfectly in balance, and that is where the power of Reiki can be of help.

THE REIKI DEGREES

The ability to bring about healing during Reiki is gained through receiving energy attunements during a special initiation ceremony. The energy attunement opens a "channel" for the universal life energy to flow through to wherever it is most needed on a physical, mental, emotional, and spiritual level.

The attunements are given by a certified Reiki Master-Teacher, and Reiki students have the opportunity to progress in their learning through three "degrees" – each one deepening and strengthening its capacity to serve as a channel for the universal life energy.

The first degree seminars generally take place over a period of two or three days, and deal mainly with the self-healing process and the recognition of one's own healing potential. Self-healing is the crucial first step in becoming a Reiki channel. Only when we take responsibility for our own healing are we in a position to support others in their healing processes.

The Reiki practitioner also understands that he or she is only a "channel." In a Reiki session, the practitioner does not direct his or her own personal energy to the recipient, but merely serves as a conduit for the universal life energy. The Reiki attunements help to cleanse and clear any obstacles that might be blocking our capacity to receive and transmit the energy – a capacity that is, in fact, natural to us all. Second and third degree trainings include learning unique Reiki symbols and their mantras, which are handed on from Reiki Master to student in confidence during the teachings. They are secret, and are therefore not published here.

CAUTION
The exercises, hand positions, and meditations described in this book are intended for the healing and harmonization of living things. The author nevertheless wishes to point out that, in the case of illness, a doctor or healing practitioner should always be consulted. The Reiki positions described may naturally be applied as an additional form of treatment.

Neither the author nor the publisher accept any responsibility for the practice or application of the methods described in this book.

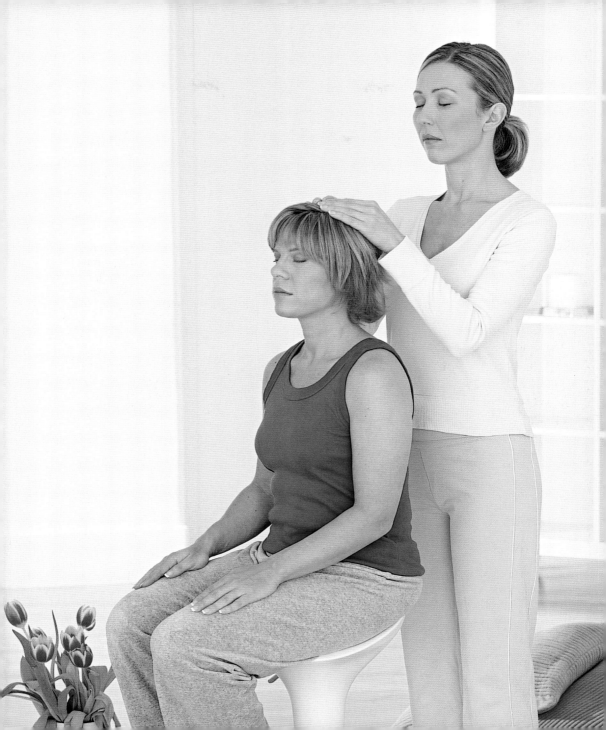

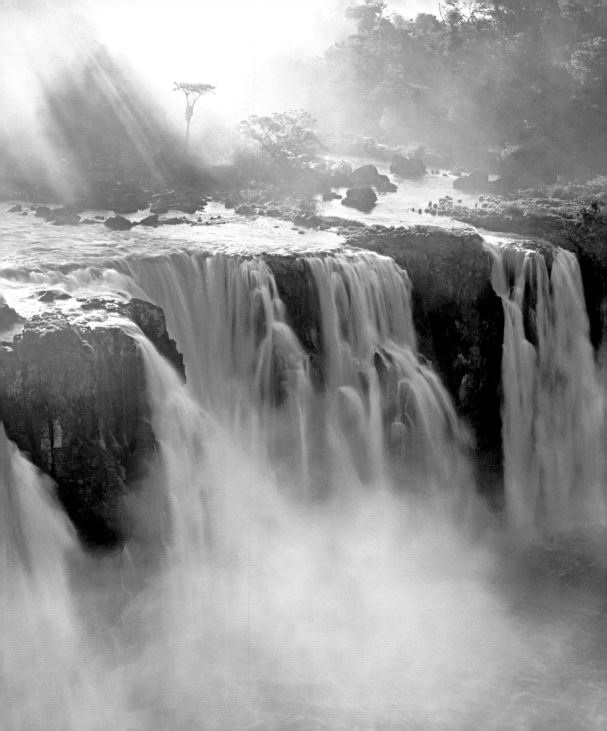

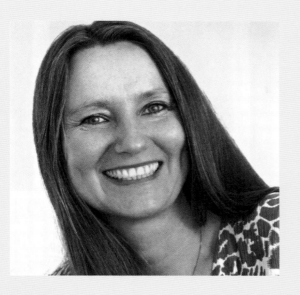

ABOUT TANMAYA
*Reiki Master-Teacher
Tanmaya Honervogt is
an author, healer, and
seminar leader. She
divides her time between
Germany and England,
and travels extensively
worldwide, giving lectures
and leading trainings.*

*Tanmaya founded the
School of Usui Reiki in 1995
in Devon, England. The
School provides a series of
certified trainings in the
traditional Usui Method.*

Those who are already familiar with Reiki will find
this book to be a handy and practical guide to some of
the basic Reiki treatments, along with many new ways
to integrate Reiki practice into your everyday life.
Those who are being introduced to Reiki for the first
time are encouraged to study the first chapter, which
goes more specifically into how Reiki works, and offers
some preliminary exercises that will help you get the
most benefit from the rest of the chapters.

I hope you enjoy reading the book and that it helps
you to find whatever support you need to bring greater
health, vitality, joy, and contentment to your life.

Tanmaya Honervogt

CHAPTER ONE

How Reiki can help you

Reiki is an ancient healing method that is easy to learn and can provide a real enrichment of your everyday life. By serving as a channel, the Reiki practitioner helps to balance and harmonize the energy of the individual, reconnecting that energy with the universal life energy that sustains us all.

Reiki can be learned by anyone who is open to it. It not only supports a sense of physical well-being, it also has a positive effect on your emotional, mental, and spiritual equilibrium. This is why after a treatment with Reiki many people feel refreshed and relaxed, clearer, and more content in themselves.

You can use Reiki to replenish your vital energy, to strengthen the immune system, and to ward off disease. At the same time, it helps in the healing of ailments and acute and chronic illnesses, from migraines to back aches, body tensions, exhaustion, depression, and fears. Reiki treats the emotional and mental causes of our discomforts, not merely the physical symptoms.

The role of a physical symptom is to show us that something is not functioning properly in the body, that our emotions are out of balance, that our mind is full of worries, or that we have been ignoring our inner spiritual needs. Reiki helps us to bring ourselves back into harmony, and at the same time to become more aware of what the body, mind, and spirit need from moment to moment throughout the day. We begin to pay more attention to small things – how we are sitting at our desks, what and how we are eating, what feelings we are experiencing, what thoughts are running through our minds – and thereby prevent them from growing into bigger things. We learn how rewarding it can be to take just a few moments to relax and revitalize ourselves, not just as a special and rare treat, but in the process of day-to-day living.

How Reiki works

Understanding how Reiki works is not difficult. All of us have experiences from our everyday lives that can give us clues. For example, we all know at least a few people who seem to make us feel better by their very presence – after spending time with them, or even just meeting them briefly on the street, we find ourselves feeling uplifted, more energetic, and happier. In contrast, there are others who, no matter what the situation, just seem to "bring us down." After interacting with them we feel drained and irritable, and even take on a dark mood – often for reasons that are difficult or impossible to identify.

Most of us have also experienced how just a thought running through the mind can bring an emotion to the surface. The memory of an argument we had with someone can recreate feelings of anger or defensiveness in the present, even though the whole incident may have happened a long time ago. Sometimes those emotions are so powerful that we feel them physically, in our bodies. When someone seems to be challenging our authority, for example, we might feel a tightness in the solar plexus. When we are frightened, we experience the fear not only in the quickening of the pulse, but also deep in the pit of the belly.

Eastern esoteric wisdom offers us a way to understand these mysteries of energy and feelings, and to use that understanding in order to heal and balance ourselves.

HOW REIKI SUPPORTS HEALTH AND WELL-BEING

- *Balances the organs and glands and their bodily functions.*
- *Releases blocks and suppressed feelings.*
- *Promotes natural self-healing.*
- *Adapts to your own natural needs.*
- *Balances the energies in the body.*
- *Enhances personal awareness and helps meditative states.*
- *Reduces and relieves stress.*
- *Promotes creativity.*
- *Strengthens life-force energy.*
- *Strengthens intuition.*
- *Treats the symptoms and causes of illness.*
- *Heals holistically.*
- *Strengthens the immune system.*
- *Relieves pain and stress.*
- *Clears toxins.*
- *Helps and soothes chronic illnesses.*
- *Always supports the healing process.*
- *Can be combined with other complementary therapies, such as acupuncture and aromatherapy.*

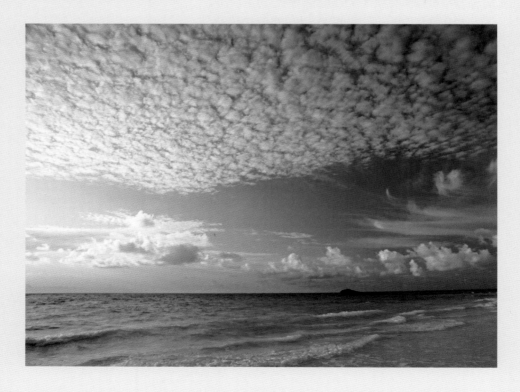

The human energy field

Every living organism pulsates with energy and is surrounded by an electromagnetic field known as an "aura." You might have seen Kirlian photographs, taken with a special camera, that actually capture a portion of this electromagnetic field on film. These photographs may be used by some complementary health practitioners to identify and diagnose physical disturbances in the body, weeks or even months before people begin to manifest symptoms. Psychics, complementary health practitioners, and healers believe that the aura contains a lot of information and, to the extent that we can learn to read it and be sensitive to it, we can know a lot about an individual's state of health and well-being.

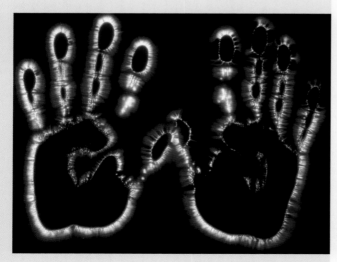

KIRLIAN IMAGERY
This Kirlian photograph shows the electromagnetic discharge surrounding a person's hands. The shape, color, and form of the discharge is said to represent a body's aura, which is indicative of physical and mental health. Although this practice is not supported by conventional medicine, some therapists claim to be able to repair damaged auras and to diagnose diseases before physical symptoms appear.

The healthy and balanced human aura extends out from the entire physical body about as far as a person's outstretched arms. Hence our tendency to want to keep people "at arms' length" if we dislike or mistrust them. In fact, we are incredibly sensitive to the "vibrations" around us, whether they come from a fellow human or whether they are emanating from an animal or a forest full of trees.

That same sensitivity that urges us to keep someone at arms' length if we feel he or she is harmful to us responds very differently when we are in the company of someone we love and trust. When we are relaxed and at ease, we find it easy – even pleasurable and nourishing – to allow the other person's energy field to meet and merge with our own. And as a by-product, the more open and relaxed we are, the more we are open to receiving the healing and revitalizing life energy that is available to nourish us all.

Many researchers believe that children, before they are taught and conditioned in the ways of the world, are naturally able to see auras. This would explain why babies are sometimes inexplicably delighted and drawn to a stranger, or equally inexplicably repelled by your favorite aunt. Something in that stranger's aura must be full of light and shiny and attractive. And your dear old aunt's nasty streak, while perhaps successfully hidden from you, is clearly visible to the child's fresh and innocent eyes.

Later in this chapter, we explore an exercise that can help you begin to experience and feel your own aura (see pages 30–1).

Chakras and the endocrine system

The hand positions that are used in Reiki are all related to the body's endocrine system and to the seven chakras, or energy centers, identified by the Eastern esoteric sciences. The endocrine system regulates hormone balance and metabolism, supplying hormones to the various organs of the body and maintaining its physical vitality. As the illustration opposite shows, the endocrine glands correspond to specific energy centers, each of which reflects an aspect of personal growth and integration.

The word *chakra* comes from the Sanskrit, meaning "wheel." This is because they appear to those who can see them as spinning energy vortices, or colored chalices of light that differ in size and activity from one individual to another. The seven chakras collect subtle energy, transform it, and supply it to associated organs and parts of the physical body.

When you treat yourself using Reiki techniques, you are in fact channeling the universal life force through the body's different chakras, helping to bring harmony to their functioning.

Many people, for example, have an excess of energy in the upper chakras and not so much in the lower chakras. We call such people "flighty" or "ungrounded." They might chatter too much, engage in restless activity, or have trouble focusing on tasks. Others might have so much of their energy concentrated in the lower chakras that they have become suspicious and fearful, self-centered and careless of the feelings of others. Or they may be so preoccupied with survival that they are unable to enjoy the higher things of life.

Many of us over the years have been conditioned by our social or religious upbringing as to condemn certain aspects of ourselves or our bodies, and if we still carry these conditionings around with us, the corresponding chakras will be out of balance. Through Reiki you can help restore this balance to a more natural state.

HOW THE SYSTEMS LINK

Each chakra is "linked" with a certain organ and region of the body and has an influence on its function. The hormones produced by the glands flow directly into the bloodstream or into the blood vessels of the organs, bringing vital energy into the body. The endocrine system supplies power to the chakras and leads the subtle energies back into the body.

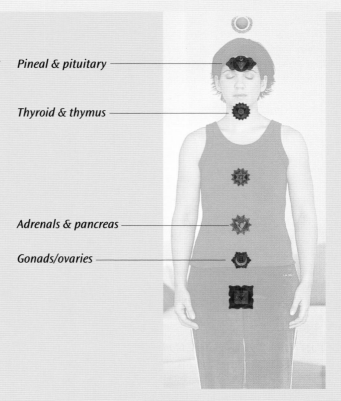

Pineal & pituitary

Thyroid & thymus

Adrenals & pancreas

Gonads/ovaries

THE SEVEN CHAKRAS

Crown (7th) – Upper brain, right eye, pineal gland. Consciousness of oneness, spiritual awareness, wisdom, intuition, realization of the higher self, all-embracing love.

Third Eye (6th) – Lower brain, left eye, nose, spine, ears, pituitary gland. Clairvoyance, telepathy, self-directedness, clarity of vision, inner understanding, inspiration, spiritual awakening.

Throat (5th) – Throat, thyroid gland, upper lungs and arms, digestive tract. Self-expression, communication, creativity, sense of responsibility.

Heart (4th) – Heart, lungs, circulatory system, thymus gland. Center of the emotions, love for self and others, peace, empathy, forgiveness, trust, spiritual development.

Solar Plexus (3rd) – Stomach, liver, gall bladder, pancreas, solar plexus. Power, strength, courage, assertiveness.

Sacral (2nd) – Reproductive organs, urogenital system, kidneys, gonads, legs. Vitality, enjoyment of life, self-esteem, relationships, desire.

Root (1st) – Adrenal glands, bladder, genitals, spine. The will to live, life force, fertility, procreation, survival.

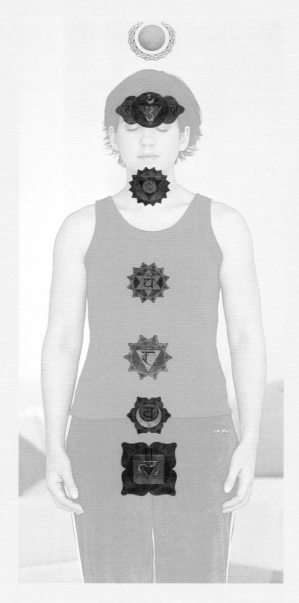

Strengthening the life force

On a physical level, Reiki helps to strengthen and sustain the body's immune system. The body is thus better able to defend itself against the effects of environmental pollution and contagious diseases. The kidneys, liver, and digestive organs are better able to deal with the toxins they encounter and flush them out of the body. And the increased awareness that Reiki brings helps us to make whatever changes in our lifestyles that are needed in order to support more relaxation and joy, which are both essential components of our health.

In addition to restoring our physical energy, Reiki also helps us to bring love and light into the dark places within ourselves, and to acknowledge and accept what we find there. When the chakras are restored to their full potential and power, each one supports all the others, and in this way we can enjoy all the pleasures that life has to offer. We experience compassion for ourselves and for other people; our words and actions have more purpose and power; and our vision is clear.

Reducing and relieving stress

Not all stress is bad – sometimes a little bit of pressure is exactly what we need in order to focus our energies, make decisions, and move out of a situation that is not supporting our growth and well-being. But when we are subjected to ongoing, chronic stress, and we do not or cannot take steps to relieve it, we can develop physical symptoms. These include ailments such as headaches, stomach aches, frequent colds, kidney pains, or general digestive disorders. These symptoms are the expression of excessive negative stress together with an imbalance of the energy system. And to relieve these symptoms, our energy needs to be restored.

Reiki techniques can help to restore and balance the energies in the body, which in turn helps us to let go and relax. This leads on to a reduction in stress, allowing us to feel more vital and alive. At the same time, Reiki supports the development of more positive responses to stressful situations so that we can deal with them more effectively and prevent them from escalating. In other words, not only the symptoms of stress, but also the causes of the problem, can be healed by using Reiki. Reiki techniques are safe and natural, and can be used together with other healing methods, including allopathy.

Reiki and meditation

Reiki prepares you for meditation, relaxing the body, mind, and emotions. Meditation also deepens the experience of Reiki. Both of them bring us into contact with the higher self, which we may or may not normally be in touch with. When we are in touch with the higher self, we know and see things more clearly. As a result, we are better able to navigate the difficult and challenging periods in life, such as changing jobs, moving to a new home, or entering into or ending a relationship. To connect to the higher self and be open to its guidance is to receive clarity, inspiration, and the courage to make the right decisions.

In addition to traditional meditation techniques such as yoga and silent sitting methods like Vipassana and Zazen, the contemporary mystic Osho has developed active meditations that include a period of physical activity and catharsis to release tensions in the physical and emotional bodies. These techniques are particularly useful for people whose work and daily activities are mostly mental and sedentary, and some of those are included in this book. These active meditations offer numerous benefits on their own, and many practitioners of traditional techniques find that the active meditations support the passive techniques, too. When the body, mind, and emotions have been cleansed of tension through active meditations, sitting silently becomes much easier.

Enhancing self-awareness, creativity, and intuition

If you are a healthy person then Reiki is great for relaxation, relieving stress, strengthening the immune system, and restoring your personal energy. It also helps your intuition to become sharper. Through Reiki you gain access to the potential that is buried within you. Each and every individual is capable of self-healing and Reiki is a wonderful creative tool with which to access this ability.

As we become more sensitive and attuned to the subtle energies within and around us, we also find that meditation becomes easier and goes more deeply. This, in turn, opens us to greater creativity in all that we do. As all great creators tell us, their finest work seems to come not from the rational, logical mind, but from a source above and beyond. They feel as though they have functioned like a "channel" for some universal source of creativity, rather than having actually created something themselves.

This ability to function as a channel is precisely what Reiki develops in aspiring practitioners, and the more we use and encourage it, the more it spreads throughout and enriches every aspect of our lives.

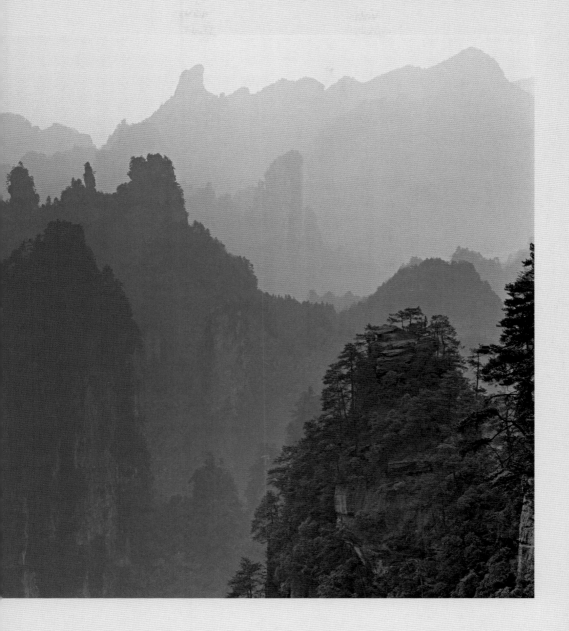

Reiki breathing exercise

This simple exercise will help you to get started with Reiki and to experience what it feels like to work with the subtle energies that have been discussed in this chapter. You can do it at any time of the day when you have just a few moments to take a little break and "come back to yourself."

   In this and all Reiki treatments, your hands are held slightly cupped, without exerting pressure, and with the fingers closed and relaxed. While treating yourself, your hands may become hot and start to tingle or throb. Don't worry, these are natural reactions. When you touch places on your body that feel hot or cold, it is likely that you have found the source of a problem; a chronic or acute disorder may well be centered there. Keep your hands on these places until you sense that the energy flow has normalized; simply use your intuition to judge when this occurs.

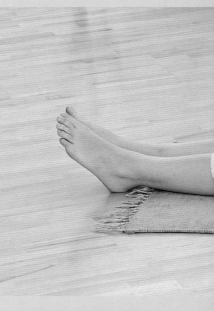

AT THE START OF EACH DAY
- *Find a comfortable position, either sitting or lying down on your back. Close your eyes. Turn your attention to your breathing, following its rhythm as it goes in and out.*

- *Turn your attention to your body and see if there are any places that feel tense or uncomfortable. Use your intuition and*

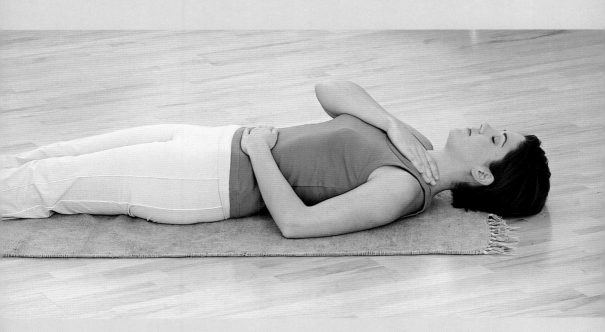

your sensitivity to identify the spot where relaxation is most needed, and place your hands there.

■ Now direct your breath consciously and repeatedly to the place where your hands are resting. Imagine that your breath is the universal life energy that flows through you. Let it collect and expand under your hands. Notice how a feeling of relaxation and peace gradually spreads from that place beneath

your hands throughout your whole body.

■ After about 5 minutes, place your hands on another part of your body, and continue the conscious breathing and visualization. You may find that your breath changes in this new position, as memories and experiences that are stored in your body begin to awaken. It is not necessary to probe consciously your feelings or to initiate

stronger breathing. Just allow yourself to let go and plunge into this feeling of flowing.

■ Repeat the exercise for two more places on the body, charging them with energy.

■ Slowly open your eyes, stretch yourself, and return to your normal daytime consciousness. You will feel more relaxed, calmer, and more centered.

Exercise to feel the aura

Earlier in the chapter we talked about the human aura, how it functions, and how healers can learn to "read" the aura to gain information about a person's state of health and well-being. Many of the Reiki hand positions are directly related to the chakras, which function as openings for energy to flow in and out of the aura, as well as into and out of the physical body. This exercise helps you to tune in to your own energy field, and become more aware of your own aura, or electromagnetic field. As you work at this exercise you will notice certain sensations flowing between the fingers and palms of your hands.

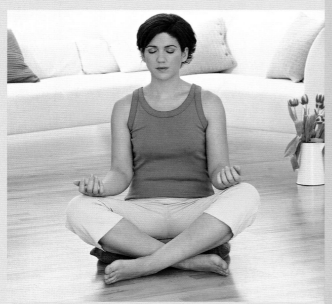

TUNING IN TO YOUR ENERGY FIELD
(01) Sit on a chair or on a cushion on the floor. Close your eyes for a few moments and then take three deep breaths, relaxing your shoulders with each exhale. At the same time, allow yourself to let go of your thoughts and preoccupations and any other tensions in your body.

(02) Now, with your arms relaxed and elbows bent, hold your hands in front of you and relax them, palms slightly cupped and facing each other, resting on your thighs. Your hands should be about 12in apart. Relax and breathe naturally, allowing your belly to rise and fall with each inhale and exhale. With closed eyes, watch from inside as the energy builds up about your two hands. Do this for between 2 and 5 minutes.

Now slowly move your hands toward each other, noticing the space between them. Become aware of the energy field between your hands as they move together; you will feel resistance.

(03) Play with the space between your hands, bringing them closer together and moving them further apart. Notice any of the sensations that you feel in your hands. You might get a feeling of tingling and pressure, increased warmth or a tickling sensation, like static electricity.

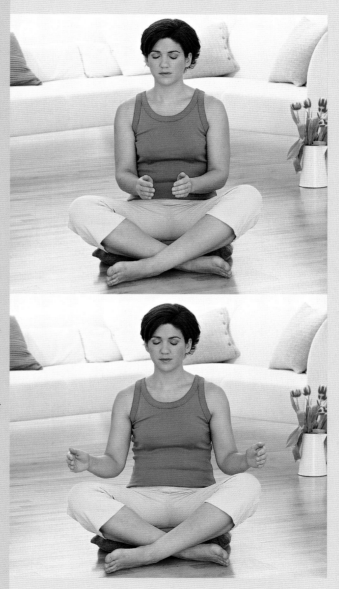

CHAPTER TWO

Let Reiki start your day

Each morning when you wake up, leaving the world of sleep and dreams, is an opportunity to reconnect with the world around you with renewed energy and a fresh perspective. Reiki supports your energy and your perspective on life, and giving yourself a Reiki treatment is an ideal way to begin each new day.

Most spiritual traditions have special times in their daily disciplines for prayer and meditation. In India, the word *sandhya* is used both for prayer and for the times of day between daylight and darkness, at sunrise and sunset. In the twilight of evening, much of nature is preparing for rest. The birds return to their chosen trees for the night, many flowers close their petals, and a palpable silence begins to descend. Thus, twilight is a particularly good time for meditations that help us to let go of the day's activities and move into silence and rest.

The silence of the night is most profound in the early morning, just before sunrise. That is why the monks and nuns of many traditions wake before dawn to begin their prayers and meditations. To begin a meditation in this atmosphere of silence and peace, and to continue as nature is touched by the rays of the rising sun and begins to wake up, brings an experience that is very different from meditations at sunset. We are swept along by a gentle tide of awakening energy that reconnects us with all the joy and vitality of life.

Which side of the bed?

The first few moments of each day are obviously important; otherwise, why should we have a saying in nearly every language that attempts to explain our all-too-common grumpiness or irritability with the excuse that we "got up on the wrong side of the bed"? The exercises and meditations in this chapter are designed to help you get up on the right side of the bed each morning. Whether you are a stay-at-home parent or an investment banker, whether your work is primarily physical and active, or sedentary and mental, you will find something here to prepare you for the demands of the day ahead.

Maybe you are the sort of person who jumps out of bed full of energy and ready to take the world by storm – if so, you will probably enjoy the Laughter Meditation (see pages 44–5) or the Nonsense Meditation (see pages 39–41). If, however, you are more the sort who enjoys taking a long time to come back into the waking world, and your first impulse when you switch off the alarm is to pull the blankets up over your head and go back to sleep, you can use the time you might have spent snoozing to give yourself a chakra-balancing treatment (see pages 36–8), or try the Heart of Peacefulness exercise (see pages 42-3). You can do both of them without even having to sit up.

Regardless of your "type," you can experiment with all the exercises to see which ones suit you best. Your preferences might change over time, or even from day to day, depending on how you are feeling or the nature of the day you are about to begin.

SANDHYA

The Indian word sandhya *is used both for prayer and for the times of day when the sun is low on the horizon – at sunrise and sunset (see right). The stillness and quiet of twilight are particularly favorable for meditations designed to help you let go of the day's activities.*

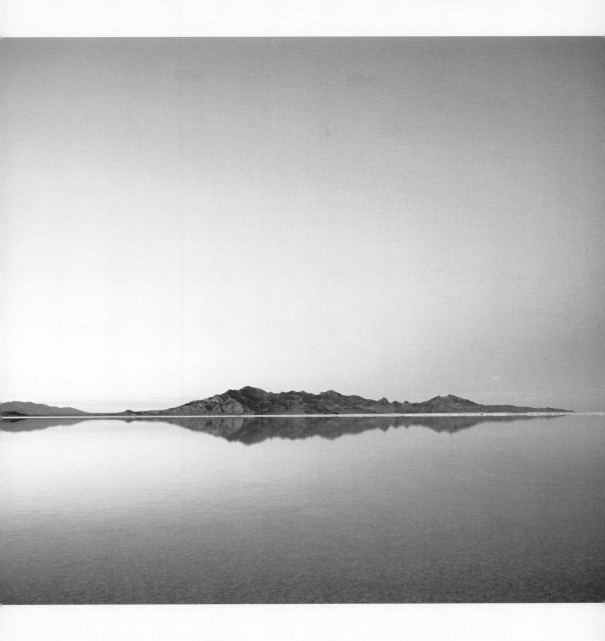

Chakra balancing

Starting your routine each morning with a chakra-balancing treatment is a great way to "stay in shape" – both physically and spiritually – even when life is better than you ever imagined it could be. If, however, you have been feeling generally out of it, or you have been experiencing low energy levels or mood swings, a chakra-balancing treatment will help bring light to problem areas. This will help you see what you need to do in order to bring yourself back into balance.

If you have had a restless night or disturbing dreams, a chakra-balancing treatment will help you let go of any residue and start afresh with the new day.

MORNING EXERCISE
(01) Lie flat with your head resting comfortably on pillows and with your legs together. Place one hand on your forehead (6th chakra) and the other over your pubic bone (1st chakra). Let your hands rest here for about 5 minutes, or until you sense that the energy is flowing equally in both places. Balancing the energy of the head and lower part of the body helps you to calm your mind and get in touch with your sexual vitality and life energy.

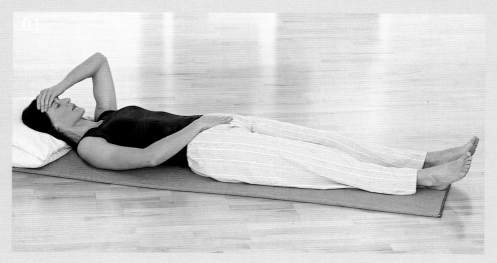

(02) Lay one hand over your throat (5th chakra) and the other on your belly (2nd chakra) below the navel. This helps to balance and harmonize the emotions and desires, and to be able to express them more easily in a creative way. Let your hands rest here for about 5 minutes.

(03) Place one hand on the middle of the chest (4th chakra) and the other on the solar plexus (3rd chakra). The 4th, or heart chakra, is the seat of our capacity for love and compassion, and the solar plexus connects us with our own source of strength and power. When these two centers are balanced, we are able to bring both love and understanding to our decisions and actions. Let your hands rest here for about 5 minutes.

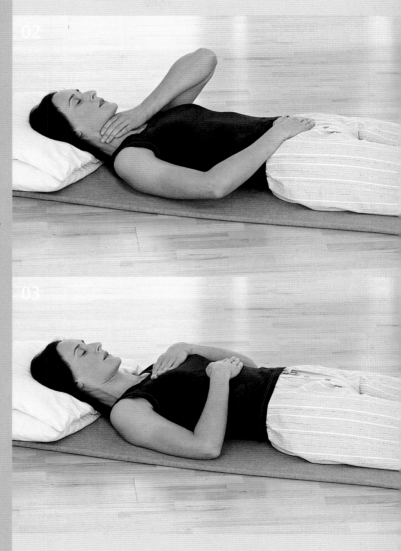

(04) Place one hand on the belly at your navel (2nd chakra) and the other on the forehead, over the third eye (6th chakra). This position will relax you deeply and allow you to let go of thoughts and feelings, promoting clarity and allowing you to see and accept what is. Let your hands rest in place for about 5 minutes.

(05) After you have balanced all your chakras, move your body gently, wiggle your toes and fingers, and stretch your whole body. Come back to normal consciousness.

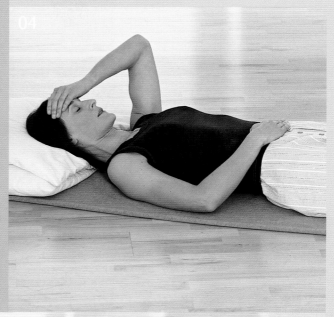

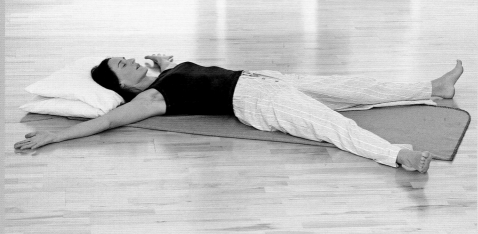

Nonsense Meditation

The mind is a miraculous mechanism that works for us tirelessly, non-stop, day after day. It analyzes and dissects, categorizes and sorts, and stores and retrieves enormous amounts of information so that we can use it when it is required. However, particularly in the modern age, as we are bombarded with ever-increasing amounts of information and imagery, the mind can become overwhelmed and fatigued by the sheer volume of input. When this occurs, we can begin to feel clouded and confused, even paralyzed by the sheer chaos of the chatter inside our brains. The information-retrieval systems of the brain can no longer function efficiently, and so we start to forget things.

When the brain is overworked and overtired, our sleep can be affected, too. Without enough time in the day to process all the information that has been given to it, the mind makes an effort to stay awake and work through the night. Even if the body can manage to fall asleep despite the ongoing activity, the quality of the rest will be inadequate, and we will wake up feeling almost as if we had not slept at all.

One of the benefits of meditation is that it gives us the ability to switch off the mind and give it a rest. For many of us, the idea of "switching off the mind" is frightening, because we identify so closely with our thoughts. Our culture has adopted Descartes' famous statement "I think, therefore I am" to an extreme degree. We think so much in the course of our every-day lives that we begin to feel that without our thoughts we would not exist at all.

The mind is just a tool to help us function and communicate. And just as our legs can be used to walk but don't need to move while we are sitting down, the mind does not need to work all the time. By giving it a chance to rest, we need not fear that we will damage its function. On the contrary, rest will help the mind to become fresher, clearer, and better able to perform the duties it was designed to do.

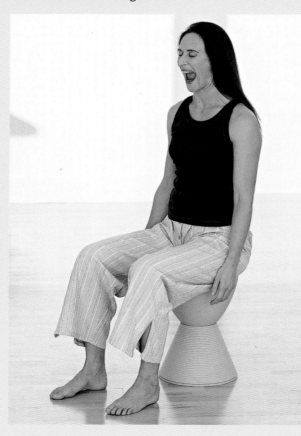

FIRST STAGE

(01) This takes 15 minutes. Sit or stand comfortably and close your eyes. Begin to blurt out nonsense words or sounds, and allow them to come out however they want. Sing, cry, shout, talk, whisper, mumble, however the sounds want to emerge. Speak any language that you don't know. If you know English, speak Chinese or Dutch; if you know French, speak Hindi or Afrikaans. If you find it difficult to begin, start with "la-la-la-di-da" and keep going until the sounds become freer and more expressive.

At the same time, allow your body to express whatever it needs to express. You might find yourself shaking your arms, jumping, kicking, standing up if you are sitting down, or lying down if you are standing up. You can have your eyes open just enough to make sure you don't bump into something and hurt yourself.

In allowing the mind to empty out the rubbish, you are giving it a shower of fresh energy so that it can function at its best throughout the day ahead.

The Nonsense Meditation is a great house-cleaning exercise for the mind. In the evening, you can use it to prepare for one of the silent meditations where "switching off" the mind is the object. In the morning, it's a good way to start the day when your list of things to do has grown so large that you find yourself paralyzed or totally immobilized by the sheer number of different items on the agenda.

The "to-do" list might include tasks that are specific to your work, problems you are having with other people that you know you must sort out, social obligations you have taken on (perhaps a little unwisely), or a combination of all these things. This little meditation will not necessarily remove any of the items from your list (although it might, simply by making space for clarity about what is really important), but it will help you clear away the static and worry that makes you feel so overwhelmed and

SECOND STAGE

(02) This stage also takes 15 minutes. Lie down on your front and feel your body sinking into the floor or mattress beneath you. This will harmonize and settle any energies and emotions that have been brought to the surface in the first stage.

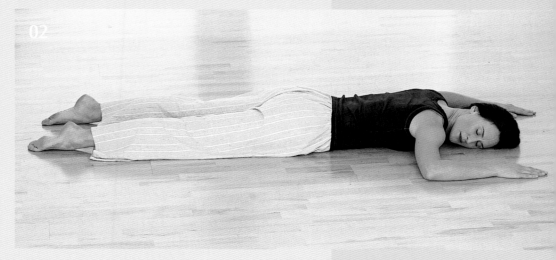

02

Heart of Peacefulness

When we are in contact with our heart it is also easier for us to come into contact with our being, or essence. Our society tends to overvalue the mind, and to regard the heart as slightly dangerous – too impulsive and irrational to be trusted. What we fail to realize is that when any of our natural energy is suppressed, that energy will find some other way to express itself. The nature of energy is to move and flow and, like water, it will find its way around any obstacle.

The problem is that when the natural flow of energy is obstructed by unnatural constraints, it tends to express itself in distorted ways. The energy that is meant to express itself as compassion and acceptance of others can become a tendency to anger, and to judge others as unworthy of our love. If our social conditioning leads us to believe that we have a duty to "love our neighbors," regardless of whether or not we actually enjoy their company, we become hypocrites – pleasant to their faces, but gossiping about them behind their backs. Our love can become possessive and jealous, our sexuality can be tainted with guilt, and our natural sense of strength and vitality can become a desire to dominate others.

Both Reiki and meditation help us to restore harmony and balance to all our energies, allowing us to express them in natural ways.

The Heart of Peacefulness is particularly good when you are having trouble staying calm and centered in the middle of difficult circumstances. If you are prone to emotional upsets and mood swings, this exercise will help you to accept and transform your negative emotions rather than trying to suppress them, leaving you with a greater sense of vitality and joy. When your mind is worried about what the day ahead might bring, it will help you to get in touch with your clarity and intuition so that you can respond more creatively to circumstances as they arise. It is also good for any difficulties you might experience falling asleep at the end of a particularly stressful day. Taking the time to connect with the natural peace that is always available to us when we are in contact with the heart brings a deep relaxation and sense of well-being.

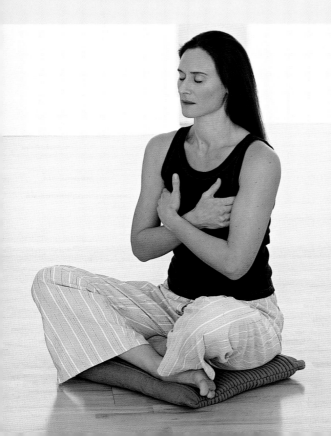

THE MEDITATION

- *Sit comfortably, or lie down and relax. You can also start this exercise as soon as you begin to wake up, before you open your eyes. With eyes closed, let your breath flow naturally in and out. Now place your right hand in your left armpit, and your left hand in the right armpit. Direct your whole attention to your chest.*

- *Allow a feeling of peace to arise from your heart. Just relax and keep your attention on this feeling.*

- *When you are centered in the heart and relaxed, you will automatically come into contact with your inner peace. The heart calms and transmits harmonic vibrations, which you experience as love and peace. Remain in this position for 10–15 minutes, enjoying this feeling.*

Laughter Meditation

Medical research has shown that having a sense of humor – about ourselves and about the situations we encounter – has an extraordinarily beneficial effect on our health and well-being. It actually affects our chemistry, brain waves, and thinking. Each and every good laugh releases tension in the body and releases hormones that revitalize and refresh us to the very core. In some Zen monasteries, the monks start and end each day with laughter.

When you are in touch with your sense of humor, you can see that so many ridiculous and amusing things are happening all around you so much of the time … how can you help but laugh? When you can laugh at yourself and the situations you find yourself in, a space is created between you and your problems. What better way to prepare for the day than to start it with a deep belly laugh, for no reason at all?

Try this laughter technique for between 5 and 10 minutes at a time, with your eyes open or closed, and you may be surprised how it will change the mood of your entire day.

THE MEDITATION
Try this meditation exercise when you wake up in the morning. Before you open your eyes, stretch and arch your whole body, like a cat. After a moment or two, start to laugh. Simply lift the corners of your mouth and laugh out loud, even if you cannot think of a single reason for it. Soon you will discover that even forced laughter will stimulate the real thing, and your laughter will become quite genuine and spontaneous. Some people find that a good way to release their laughter is to lie on their backs and raise their knees up toward their chest, even kicking their legs and playing with their feet like babies do. If it helps, do it, and continue for between 5 and 10 minutes.

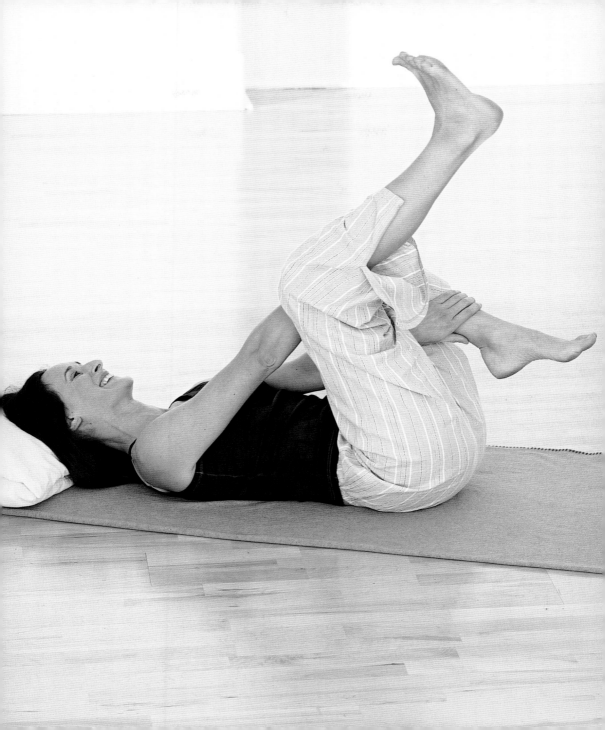

CHAPTER THREE

Traveling light with Reiki

One of the benefits of travel is that often when you are in transit, you have a little extra spare time on your hands to play with. And one of the benefits of Reiki is that you can take it with you no matter where you go – and it doesn't take up any space in your bag.

Most people find that modern-day travel is stressful to some degree. Whether we find ourselves strap-hanging on a crowded bus or commuter train, sitting in a traffic jam on some anonymous motorway, or racking up the frequent-flier miles on endless business trips, we tend to end up frazzled more often than we find opportunities to enjoy the scenery along the way. Instead of using that time wishing you had already arrived at your destination, why not use it for relaxation and healing?

Long-distance travel brings its own special challenges, including changes of time zone and climate. It is important to give your immune system and all the subtle rhythms of the body as much support as you can, and Reiki offers many treatments to do just that. When you reach your destination, use any extra time you might have available to give yourself a full self-treatment. It will help you to avoid the feelings of tiredness and disorientation that are otherwise common when traveling by jet.

The following pages contain useful meditations and treatments, both for your ordinary daily commute and for those longer business or recreational trips.

Bon voyage!

Reiki on the move

Whether you are traveling on a train, bus, or plane, there is a range of Reiki self-treatments you can try right where you are sitting. You should choose the particular treatment according to any physical, emotional, or mental issues you are dealing with at the time and that could benefit from a little extra attention. Although the positions here are numbered, you don't have to use them in any particular sequence or combination.

FRONT POSITION ONE
Place your fingers just below the collarbone as shown (below far left) for Front Position One. This is ideal for strengthening your immunity and stimulating lymph circulation, both of which are beneficial when you are traveling with other people.

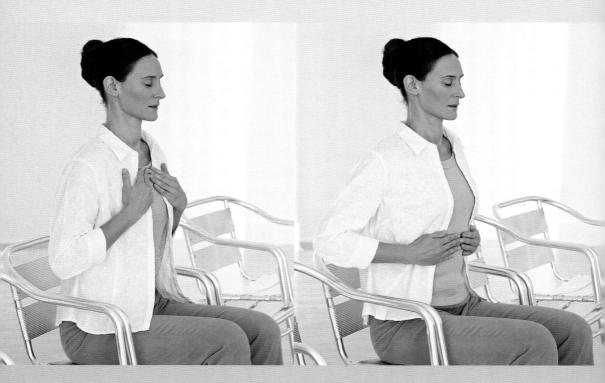

FRONT POSITIONS TWO AND THREE

If you are having trouble with digestion, Front Positions Two (below left) and Three (below) are easy to do while sitting down anywhere when traveling. Both positions are also good for supporting self-confidence and easing fears.

HEAD POSITION FIVE

This position, Head Position Five (below), harmonizes blood pressure and metabolism, and also promotes self-expression. Make sure that your wrists are touching in the center of your throat.

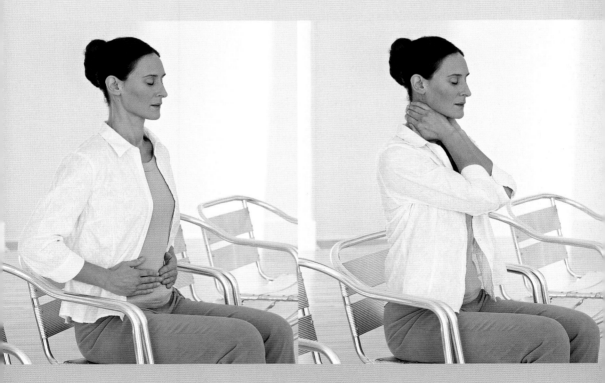

Our protective aura

We are sometimes affected by the moods and thoughts of others without knowing it, particularly if we are very sensitive. If we don't know how to protect ourselves and stay in contact with our own center as people around us are unconsciously broadcasting their thoughts, tensions, and problems, we can even start thinking those thoughts and problems are our own.

Our own subtle energies are constantly affecting, and being affected by, the energies of those around us. Some of us are more sensitive and vulnerable to the effects of this constant energy exchange than others. This doesn't need to be a disturbance. When we are balanced and strong within ourselves, it is no more harmful than breathing. This visualization exercise is a help in supporting that balance and strength.

Creating a protective aura is particularly good for those whose daily routine includes riding crowded buses or commuter trains. It strengthens and supports the portion of the aura that immediately surrounds the physical body, and reinforces your physical and emotional strength. It can help you to stay centered and relaxed in yourself, even in the middle of commuter chaos. Otherwise, you could easily gather together physical tensions as the body shrinks from contact in an effort to protect you.

If you often feel unsettled or disturbed by other people's energies after being in a public place or at work, try this meditation before going to sleep at night and when you wake up in the morning. This will deepen and strengthen the effects, so that soon you will feel strong and centered wherever you go.

VISUALIZE YOUR AURA

- *Sit comfortably and close your eyes. Begin to visualize that your entire body is surrounded by an aura of golden light in the same shape as your body that extends out about 6in.*

- *Imagine that this light is protecting you, so that no tensions can penetrate it from the outside. Stay with the visualization for about 5 minutes, and then bring yourself back to normal consciousness.*

- *If you do this meditation just before you fall asleep, you can imagine the aura covering you like a blanket the whole night long. As soon as you wake up in the morning, feel the protective aura still surrounding you; rest and enjoy this feeling for a few moments before you get out of bed.*

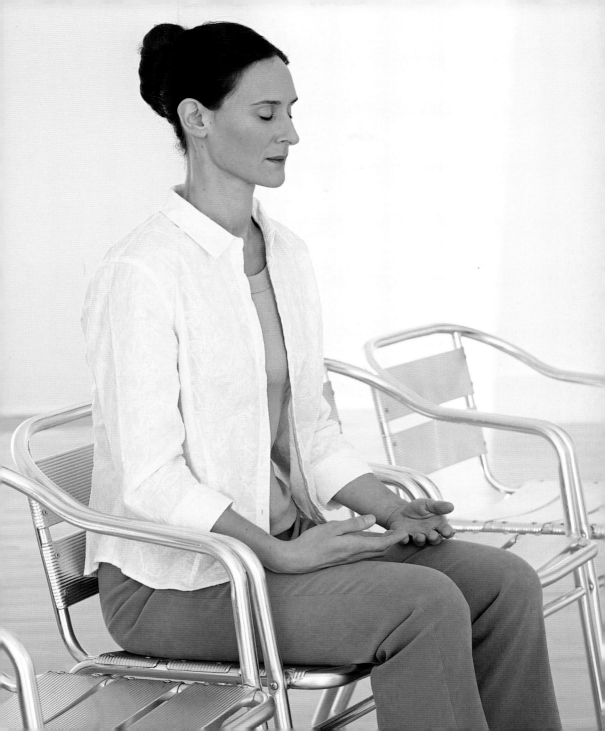

Unjamming the traffic

Planners have discovered a Catch-22 in trying to create more roads and highways to deal with ever-increasing levels of traffic. Their studies have shown that each time a road is widened or a new highway is built, the amount of traffic on it increases, and does so at such an accelerated rate that any benefit resulting from the expansion is only short-lived. Those of us who must endure a daily commute on crowded roads know this from bitter personal experience. Often it seems that we could reach our destination faster on foot than sitting behind the wheel of a car in a traffic jam. The frustration that arises when we are faced with lengthy

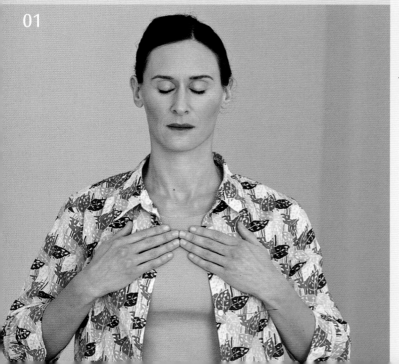

01

CALMING TREATMENT
(01) Place your hands on the left and right sides of your upper chest, with your fingers touching just below the collarbone. This position helps to get rid of negativity.

delays is only made worse when we have to suffer the noisy impatience, aggression, and "road rage" of some of our fellow drivers.

When those around you are honking their horns or shouting, it can be difficult to maintain your equilibrium. Next time you are stuck in neutral gear and need to put some distance between yourself and the ruckus, try this treatment to calm your emotions.

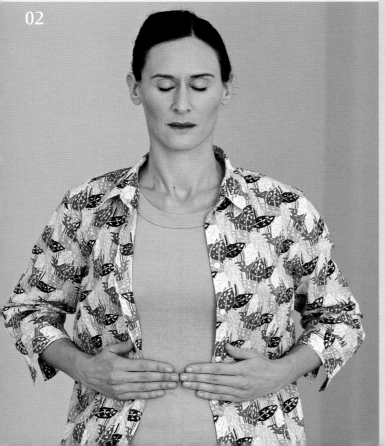

02

(02) To promote relaxation and reduce feelings of frustration, place your hands over your lower ribcage above the waist, with your fingers meeting in the middle.

Meditation and plane travel

High above the clouds, where the accustomed pull
of gravity is diminished, you may find it easier to slip
into a meditative state. This is one of the reasons why
we so often associate meditative retreats with the
Himalayan heights.

Traveling by plane can put a real strain on the body,
and it is a good idea to follow the advice given by
frequent travelers and medical authorities: drink
plenty of water during the flight, rather than
accepting the free alcoholic drinks, and eat sparingly
– take only what really appeals to you. Wear
comfortable, non-constricting clothing and shoes.
Get up and walk around as often as it is safe and
permitted to do so. And when you are confined to
your seat, try this meditation.

MEDITATIVE HIGH

- *Close your eyes and take a few moments to
  imagine that your body is expanding,
  becoming ever bigger. Allow your sense of
  your body to continue to expand until it
  fills the whole aircraft.*

- *You are growing bigger and bigger – you
  are now bigger than the aircraft, and the
  plane is inside you.*

- *Now imagine and feel that you have
  expanded into the surrounding sky ... You
  are as vast as the sky itself, and the clouds
  and stars are all moving around inside you.
  You are boundless – unlimited.*

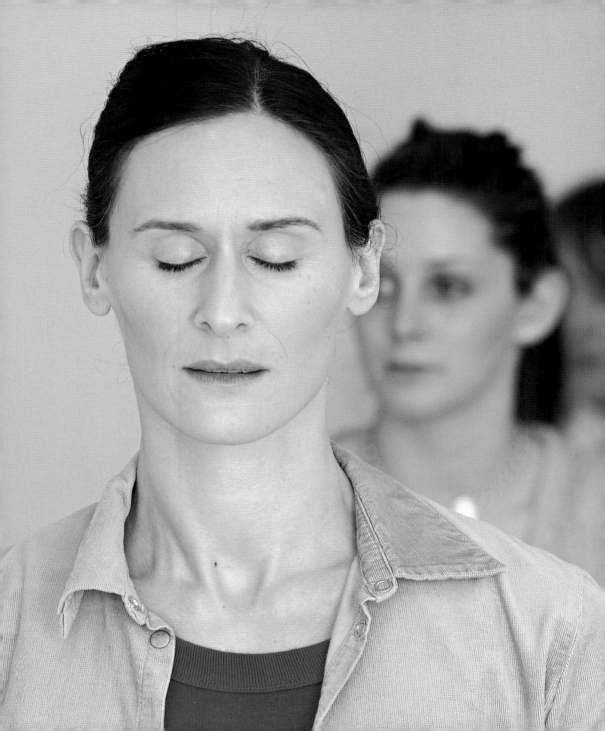

Talking to your body

Even a three-hour time zone change when traveling can disrupt our routines, especially when part of the journey also involves sleeping in unfamiliar hotel beds, eating restaurant food, and navigating unfamiliar streets. And the "jet lag" that plagues us after much longer journeys can throw our bodily systems out of whack for days.

Most people with an abundance of frequent-flier miles can tell you their favorite recipes for overcoming the effects of jet lag. Some might take melatonin supplements, while others make sure that they are awake to watch the sunset and the sunrise at their destination. Or they might advise you just to soldier on through your activities with such enthusiasm that you lose all sense of time. But regardless of how long or short the journey is, it is important to stay in touch with the needs of your body.

This exercise is good for doing just that. It is an adaptation of a "meditative therapy" developed by Osho. With practice, you can begin to learn the body's language so that you can speak to it and listen to it. Once you have truly befriended your body and learned its subtle ways of communicating, many of your everyday stress-related physical symptoms will happily disappear.

BODY–MIND BALANCING

- *Lie down or sit in a relaxed position. Then close your eyes. Now direct the light of your consciousness within your body. Look for any tensions there, moving slowly and in a relaxed way from your toes to your head.*

- *Anywhere that you feel there is tension or discomfort, talk to that part of your body as if you are talking to a friend. Create a dialogue between yourself and your body. "How are you?" … "Is there anything I can do for you?" … Then wait for an answer. The answer may not come in words; it may be an intuitive feeling or a mental image or series of images. Allow yourself to be surprised.*

- *Thank your body for being so helpful to you and taking so much care, functioning so silently and faithfully for all these years.*

■ Tell your body that it is fine to relax, and that there is nothing to fear. Wherever you feel any tensions or discomfort, acknowledge that this is your body's way of trying to help you by telling you that something needs attention. Reassure your body that you are listening to its needs, and that it is fine to drop this tension or discomfort.

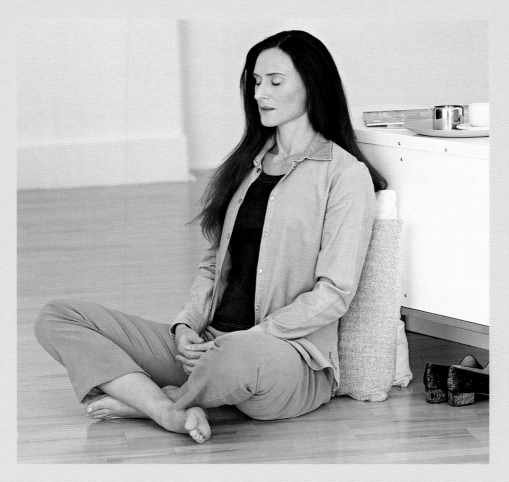

Grounding

This exercise is good any time you need to feel "down to earth," not only when traveling. Whenever you are grounded, you are connected to the earth and centered in yourself. You become one of those people who, rather than being preoccupied with thoughts and worries, seem to have "both feet on the ground." You know where you stand and can stand up for yourself when it is needed.

This exercise energizes all the chakras, balancing and harmonizing them while at the same time bringing strength and vitality to your whole organism. You can do the short form (the first four stages) or the longer form, depending on the time you have available.

ENERGIZING YOUR CHAKRAS

- *Stand comfortably, with your feet a shoulder-width apart. Close your eyes.*

- *Breathe in deeply and, as you breathe out, let your shoulders hang loose and relaxed. Repeat this 2 or 3 times, each time relaxing the tensions in your shoulders and other parts of your body on the exhale.*

- *Now turn your attention to your feet. Imagine that you are taking up energy from the earth. As you breathe in, allow earth energy to flow into your left foot. You can also imagine drawing the energy up from the center of the earth. This energy flows up your left leg and through the root (1st) chakra, low in the pelvis. Allow this chakra to relax and open to the earth below.*

- *As you breathe out, imagine earth energy flowing down your right leg and through your right foot, back into the earth. Imagine the energy flowing back to the very center of the earth. After 5 minutes or so, you can end the exercise, or you can continue to treat all the chakras as described below.*

- *In this stage, continue to imagine earth energy flowing into you through your left foot as you breathe. Drawing the energy up through your left leg, allow it to flood into the sacral (2nd) chakra. As you breathe out, allow the energy to flow back down the right leg and right foot into the earth once more. Continuing in this fashion, treat all seven chakras, including the crown, allowing earth energy to flow through each center for about 2 minutes.*

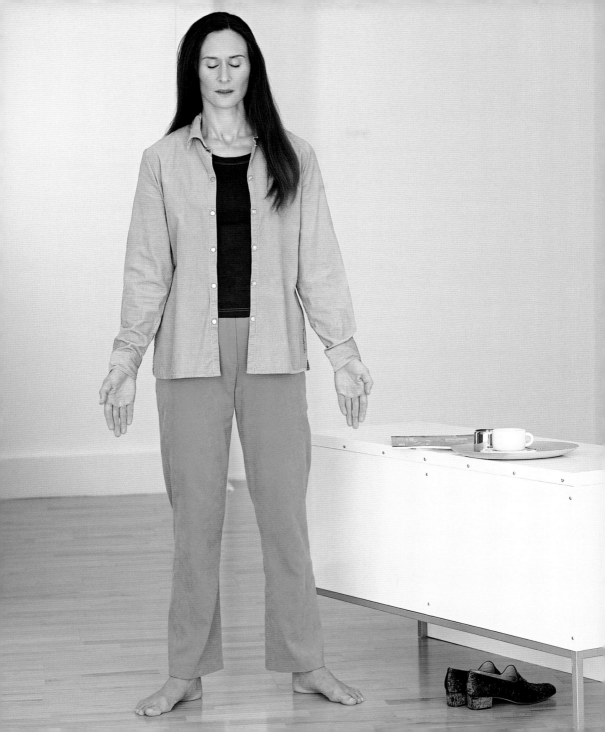

Nadabrahma Meditation

This meditation is based on an old Tibetan technique and has a powerful calming effect on the mind and body. The meditation is particularly useful to reintegrate and harmonize the subtle energies of the body that may have been disrupted by travel, and it can easily be done in your hotel room. The entire meditation lasts an hour, and there is no fixed time of day that is best, as long as you can arrange not to be disturbed for the duration. If you practice it in the morning, it is advisable to rest for about 15 minutes before starting your day's activities. This meditation is also very effective for healing, and can easily be done anywhere as long as you are able to sit up.

There are three stages to the meditation, and it may help to make a tape of a gong sounding at the correct intervals to indicate the different stages.

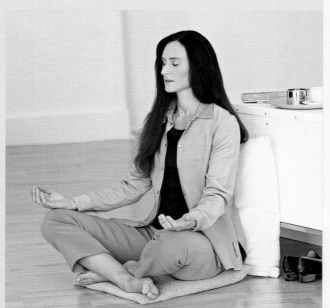

Stage 1 (30 minutes)

Sit in a relaxed position with your eyes and mouth closed. Start to hum so that you can hear yourself easily. Find a tone that allows you to feel the vibration of sound in your body, and let this vibration spread. Imagine that your body is hollow inside, like the stem of a bamboo, and is completely filled by the vibration of your humming. You can change pitch and tone from time to time, but keep the humming continuous as you breathe out.

Stage 2a (7 minutes)

At this stage, stop humming and, with your palms facing upwards, hold both hands in front of your body at the height of your navel. Begin to move them very slowly outwards and away from the body, with the hands beginning to separate as your arms are extended, making two large circles to the right and to the left. Feel as if you are gently offering

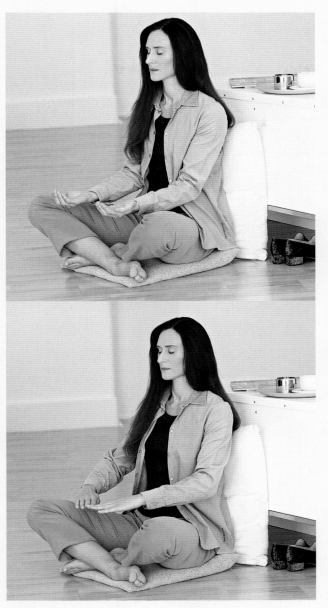

your energy to the whole universe. The movement should be so slow that it is almost imperceptible.

Stage 2b (7 minutes)
At this point turn your palms downwards, facing the earth. At the same time, reverse the direction of the circular movement, bringing your hands back in towards the navel and then separating again on both sides, continuing their circular movements in the other direction. Feel the energy of the universe coming back to and entering you now. Allow your body to sway gently if it wants to.

Stage 3 (15 minutes)
Remain sitting or lie on your back, feeling the stillness and silence within.

Sleep help

There are many factors that can make it difficult for you to fall asleep. A strange environment, jet lag, a busy mind full of worries or anxieties, or just a general restlessness and an inability of the body to get comfortable. This treatment brings comfort to the body and relaxation to the mind.

SLEEP POSITION
(01) Make yourself comfortable in your normal sleeping position, lying either on your back or on your side.

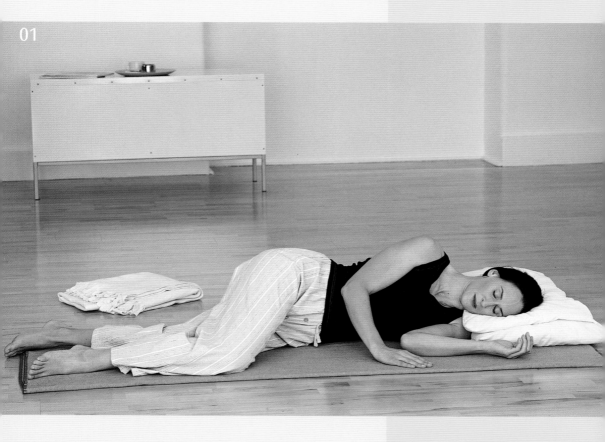

01

(02) Now place one hand on your forehead and the other on your stomach. Feel the gentle rise and fall of your stomach as you breathe in and out.

(03) Stay in this position for about 10 minutes, or for as long as you need for the Reiki energy to generate a feeling of deep relaxation. You will soon fall asleep.

02/03

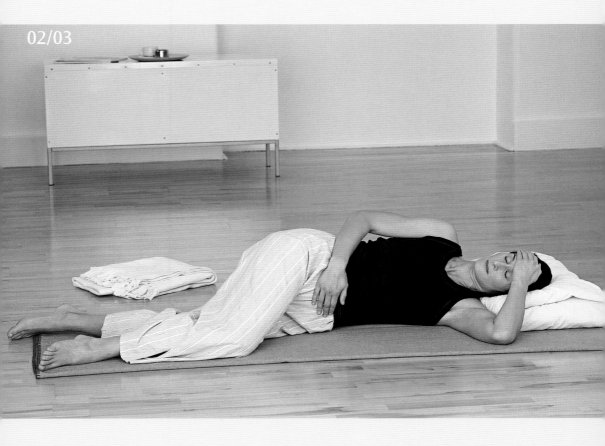

CHAPTER FOUR

Reiki at work

When we cannot cope with the demands placed on us at work, we may react with a variety of physical, emotional, and mental symptoms of stress. Reiki is a tool that we can use to respond creatively to the demands of everyday life, rather than react to them with self-defeating patterns of behavior.

Even when we love what we do for a living, most of us experience our fair share of challenges during the working day. A shift in priorities can render days of planning irrelevant; equipment breakdowns can cause us to miss deadlines; a key member of the team can fall ill, making their expert input unavailable at a critical point.

On the relationship level, "office politics" might require you to socialize with co-workers whose company you don't particularly enjoy or to keep quiet when every fiber of your being wants to speak out.

Work that involves dealing with the public requires us to treat each person we meet with courtesy and respect, even if that person is being unreasonable. If we are going through difficult times in other parts of our lives, we are expected not to allow this to affect our work. But regardless of any or all of these challenges and demands, we are expected to be able to think clearly, make the right decisions, and cooperate with others.

In this chapter, you will find a number of treatments to help you through the working day. Not everyone is fortunate enough to have a private office, or a lounge that they can retire to and give themselves a half-hour Reiki treatment. In that case, you can give yourself a full treatment once you arrive at home.

As you continue your experiments with Reiki, you will discover many things you can do for yourself during the day. Many Reiki treatments take only a few moments and do not attract much attention.

Quick work de-stresser

There are many different types of stress that can affect you while at work – an urgent deadline, a sense of being overwhelmed by the sheer quantity of things to do, or worries about whether or not you actually have the skills needed to do what is expected. This quick treatment rejuvenates body, mind, and emotions, and is very effective after lunch or in the late afternoon, when energy levels may be depleted.

For the full treatment, lie down if possible, or sit comfortably and relaxed in a chair. Cover your eyes with a blindfold or, if you are lying down, you can use a small beanbag to create a slight, relaxing pressure on the eyeballs. Hold each hand position for between 3 and 5 minutes, for a total of 15 minutes.

If it is not possible at your workplace to give yourself the full treatment, the first step is easy, unobtrusive, and effective. Or, choose one or two of the hand positions from the other steps shown here that deal most directly with the symptoms you are feeling at the time. You can also simply close your eyes and sit relaxed in your chair for the treatment.

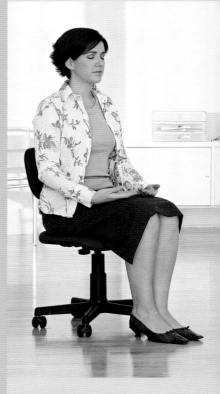

STRESS RELEASE
(01) Take a deep breath and, as you breathe out, let go of any tensions in your body and mind. Repeat this 2 or 3 times.

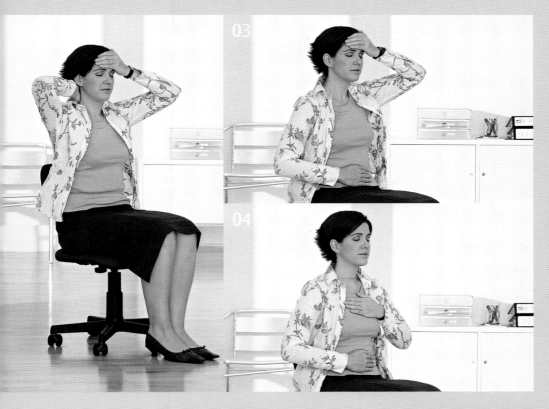

(02) If you are lying down, cup the back of your head with both hands. If you are sitting, place one hand on your forehead and the other on the back of the head, just above the neck. This position calms the mind and emotions, and relaxes the tension that can be the cause of headaches.

(03) Now lay one hand on your navel and the other on your forehead. This position has a calming and centering effect, and relaxes and harmonizes the intestines and solar plexus.

(04) Keeping one hand on your navel, move the other to the middle of your chest. This balances the energy from the heart center (4th chakra) and the sacral (2nd chakra).

Mood manager

Having emotions is part of what makes us human. We can be happy or sad, angry or full of compassion, depressed or overflowing with optimism and hope. At times those emotions are clearly related to external circumstances in our lives, and at times they seem to arise for no particular reason that we can identify. At times it is not appropriate, for one reason or another, to express our emotions. Nevertheless, the emotions and feelings do exist, and it is important that we acknowledge and accept them.

This exercise is designed to help us deal with those times when we are suffering from mood swings. It helps us to move to our own center and relax, knowing that "this, too, will pass." It is based on the following Sufi story, which gives deep insight into the ever-changing nature of the events that happen in our lives.

A king who felt frustrated with the ups and downs of life asked a Sufi mystic how to become a master of all his moods — high and low, happy and sad. The mystic gave him a ring with a secret formula carved into the band underneath the precious stone. He said to the king: "There is one condition that must be fulfilled for the secret formula to work. You should look at it only when you feel that everything is lost. Only if you are truly in your darkest hour will the secret be revealed to you." The king agreed, and some months later his country was under attack, his army had been defeated, he was utterly alone and was fleeing for his life. At the very moment the king came to a deep abyss, he remembered the ring and opened it. The message beneath the stone read, "This, too, will pass."

LIFTING A BAD MOOD

- *Sit silently and relax. Become aware of your breathing.*

- *With each exhale, allow your dark mood to leave you, melting away and dispersing, and taking all the tensions in your body with it. Do this consciously for about 5 minutes.*

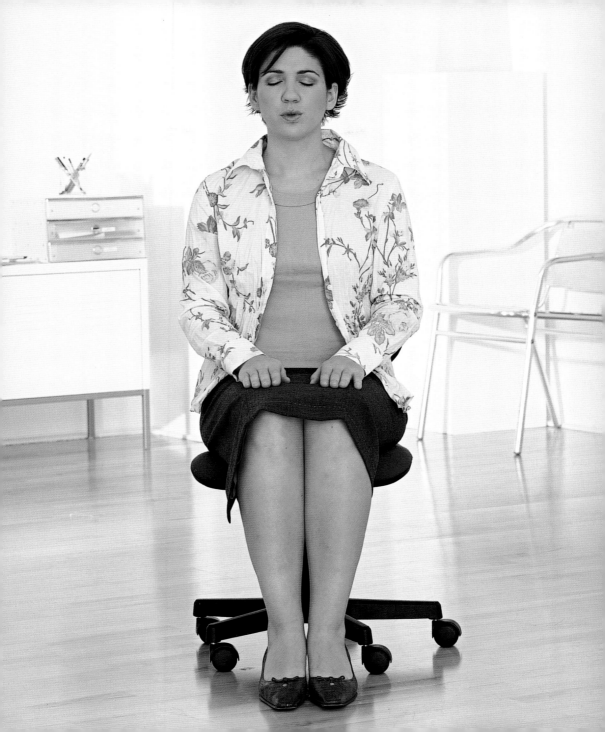

STOP!

One of the benefits of Reiki is that it brings more awareness to the subtle messages that your body sends you when it is feeling out of sorts. Chronic pain or stress-related illness does not arise just overnight. It is often the result of weeks, months, or even years spent ignoring the small signals and quiet whispers that are easy to dismiss in the course of a busy day. Depression, doctors tell us, is often accompanied by chemical imbalances in the brain – but no one is certain where the cause-and-effect relationship lies, or even if there is one. The insight of many meditators

GETTING IN TOUCH WITH YOURSELF

- *Whenever you think of it during the day – immediately, the very moment the thought arises in your mind – say "Stop!" and freeze in place. Do not move or adjust your position at all for about 30 seconds.*

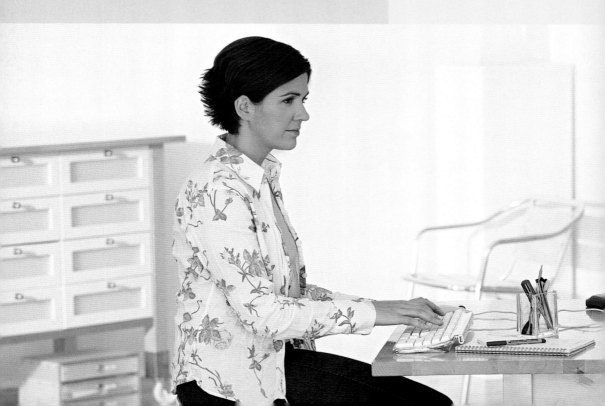

■ *Take note of your body – are your shoulders hunched? Are you slouched in your chair? Where was your mind before you said, "Stop"? Were you attentive to what you were doing, or were you daydreaming about another time and another place? How are you feeling?*

■ *Continue with what you were doing.*

and holistic healers is that depression is what happens to you if you continually deny yourself permission to express your feelings and to move in the ways you want to move.

Becoming aware of your patterns is the first step in dissolving them and becoming more spontaneous and free – on a physical, emotional, and mental level. As you become more aware, you simultaneously become more responsive to the inner guidance that tells you what you really need, and the best way to balance those needs with what is expected of you.

This exercise can help you to become aware of habitual patterns of physical behavior that contribute to chronic pain in the body. It can also help you to become aware of any self-defeating mental or emotional patterns. The secret to the exercise is to do it as thoroughly as possible and, as far as possible, to take yourself by surprise. It is very easy to integrate into your everyday activities – the more mundane and routine the activity the better. Walking down the hallway, sitting at your desk, eating your lunch, filing papers, or making your list of things to do … any small activity becomes an opportunity to STOP! and take note of what is happening in your body and mind, and how you are feeling.

Letting your worries go

Thoughts are ephemeral and fleeting, but they can nevertheless have a powerful effect on how we feel. One thing that meditators learn is how to observe thoughts as if they are clouds in the sky, or traffic passing by on the road. When we allow our thoughts to move without grasping on to them or judging them, we find that they move very quickly at first, often in somewhat quirky ways. A barking dog reminds us of the friendly little beagle owned by a childhood neighbor, which in turn leads us on a nostalgic tour of the neighborhood. We wander past the park where we gathered with friends after school, and see the group of old men who used to play chess there on Thursday afternoons. Thursday, we suddenly think, is when we have an appointment with the dentist – and our mental picture of the tray of dental instruments reminds us that we must search for our favorite pen, which we seem to have misplaced somewhere at home. And so on it goes. If we can simply sit and observe our thoughts for a longer period of time, gaps start to appear when one thought goes and another one has not come yet to take its place.

Worries happen when we get "stuck" with a thought. The kinds of thoughts that get stuck are often related to something that we fear (or hope) might happen in the future, or something that we regret has happened in the past. Nourished by our energy and attention, the thought goes around and around and around. We can't do anything about it, of course – the past can't be undone, and the future is yet to come. But although we know this, somehow we cannot let it go.

RECONNECTING WITH THE PRESENT
(01) Sit in a chair or lie down comfortably. Relax your breathing and place your hands over your eyes, resting your palms on your cheekbones. This position balances the pituitary and pineal glands, which regulate hormones in the body and affect your emotional well-being.

When you are feeling tense, tired, and worried, it is time to take a few moments to relax and reconnect with yourself. In the process, you will be reconnecting with the present moment, which is all you have. This treatment is easy to do sitting in a chair, and you can also do it lying down. It helps to relax your body and mind, allowing you to let go more easily of tensions and worries. It works on many levels to nourish you and help you feel better about yourself.

Any of the hand positions below and on the following pages can also be used individually to treat the particular symptoms described. Hold each hand position for about 3 to 5 minutes.

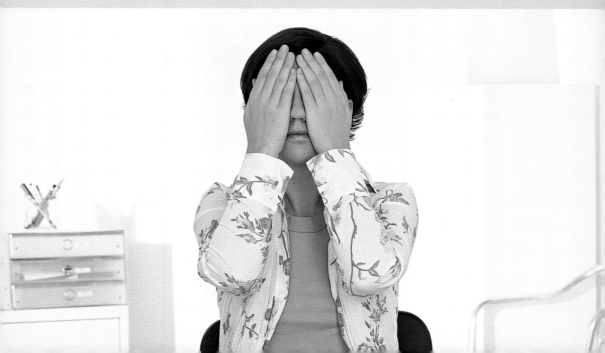

(02) Now place your hands on both sides of your head. Your fingers should be just touching at the top of your head, and the heels of your hands should be resting over your temples. This position helps to harmonize the logical/rational and the intuitive/feeling hemispheres of the brain, and relaxes and calms the conscious mind. It improves clarity of thought, memory and enjoyment of life, and eases depression.

(03) Now cup the back of your head, just above the neck, with both hands. This position relaxes the unconscious mind and calms strong emotions, such as fear, worry, anxiety, and shock. It promotes a feeling of security and helps to calm and clarify thinking.

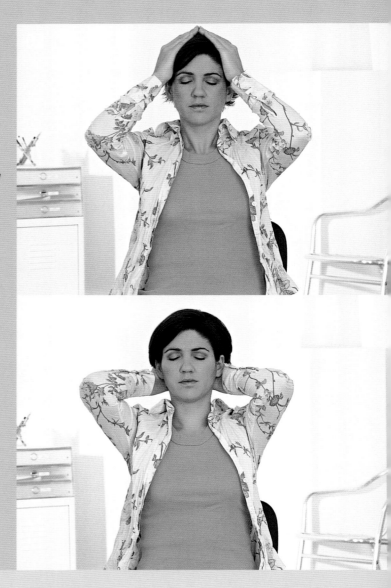

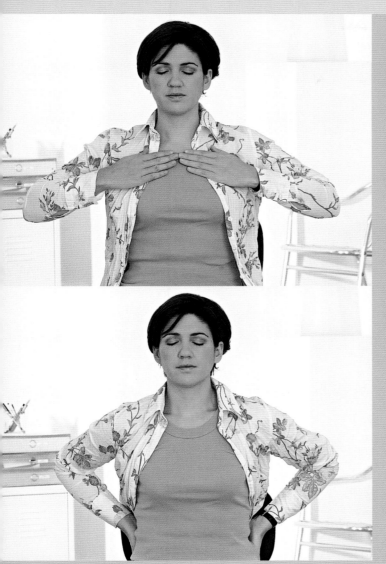

(04) *Lay your hands on the left and right side of your upper chest, fingers touching just below the collarbone. This position allows you to let go of negative emotions, especially those associated with feeling weak or depressed. It supports your capacity for love and enjoyment of life.*

(05) *Place your hands on your back at waist height, over the kidneys, fingers pointing toward the spine. This position treats the nervous system, relaxing fears and enhancing confidence. By releasing the middle back, we let go of the past and of stress and pain.*

The joy of living

The emotion of joy happens when the body, mind, and heart all function together. Joy contains pleasure and happiness, yet it is somehow more than this – an overflow of energy, love, peace, and harmony.

Most of us tend to live in our heads most of the time, and we tend to use the rational, logical side of our brain predominantly. But if we don't take time to connect with our hearts, we can end up feeling dry and lifeless. The head knows how to analyze problems

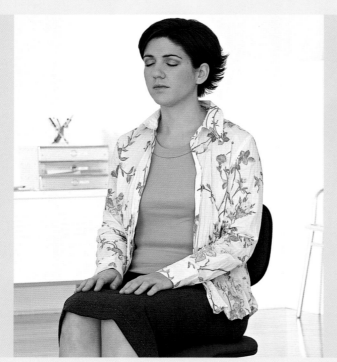

PREPARING TO MEET OTHERS
(01) Sit comfortably in a chair or lie down with your eyes closed. Place your hands loosely on your thighs and take a deep breath. As you breathe out, make a little sigh with an "aaah" sound. Relax your shoulders.

and solve them in a logical way. The heart knows how to relax, enjoy, and celebrate. Most importantly, though, the heart knows how to love, and when there is love there is also acceptance and relaxation.

Include this self-healing treatment as part of your preparation for meetings with co-workers or clients. It will bring a new quality of insight and compassion to your interactions with others.

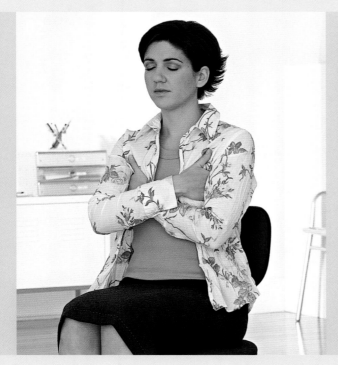

(02) Put your right hand in your left armpit and your left hand in your right armpit. Place your attention fully on the area of your chest between your armpits and allow feelings of calm, relaxation, and peace to come to the surface.

(03) Continue sitting, or lie down, and allow yourself to relax even more completely. Place your hands over your eyes, resting the heels of your hands on your cheekbones. Reiki energy affects the production of endorphins, the body's "happiness hormones." Make the sound "Yaa-hum," and allow the vibration of the sound to reach your heart. Do this for up to 5 minutes.

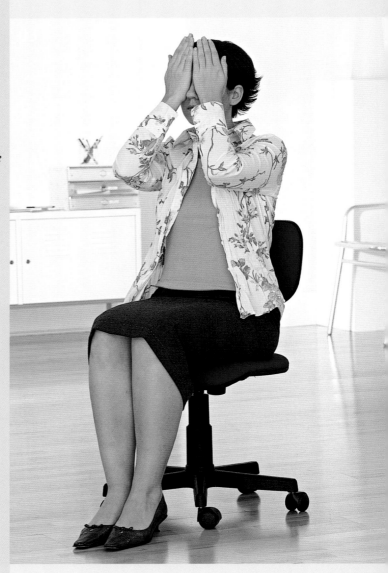

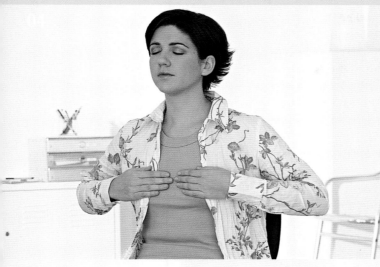

(04) Place your hands on your chest or breasts, harmonizing and balancing the male and female energies as well as the right and left side of your body.

(05) Place one hand on your navel and the other just above it. Allow the Reiki energy to expand there, grounding you and supporting your sense of inner direction. Those who have lower back problems can elevate their feet if they are lying down.

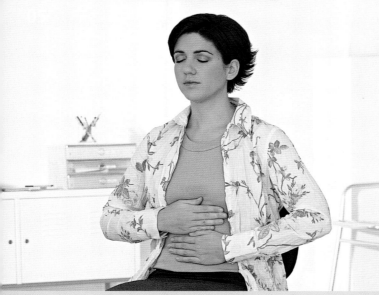

Getting your head together

If you have to give a presentation you will want your mental faculties to be functioning at their very best. In group discussions and meetings, everybody benefits when the participants can present their views clearly and concisely. The treatment presented below and on the facing page will help you to "get your head together" for mental challenges, and to ease any emotional disturbances or fears that might be hindering your capacity to think clearly. When you are feeling clear, you will find it easy to state your position, even in front of large groups of people. And when you are feeling confident and relaxed, you can turn your energy toward helping others understand rather than worrying about what they think of you, or whether you might have to defend yourself.

BEFORE A BIG MEETING
(01) Place your hands on either side of your head above the ears and touching the temples. This position harmonizes the right and left sides of the brain, bringing your intuitive and rational capacities into harmony. When the two hemispheres of the brain are balanced, you can even deal with complex issues more effectively.

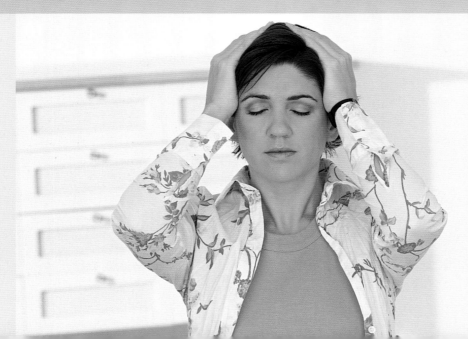

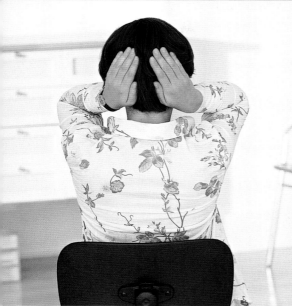 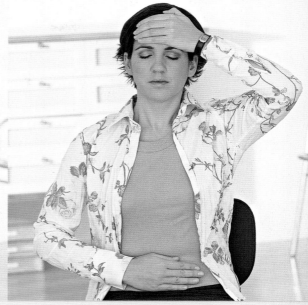

(02) Place your hands on the back of your head as if you are holding a ball in your hands. This position supports intuition, calms the mind and emotions, and eases any fears and insecurities you might be feeling.

(03) Place one hand over the solar plexus (3rd chakra) and the other on the middle of the forehead, over the third eye (6th chakra). This treatment integrates excess energy in the head with the solar plexus and it is particularly effective for those feelings of nervousness or "stage fright." When you are feeling nervous, the reason is usually because you are imagining all types of worst-case scenarios, and frightening yourself as a result. This chakra-balancing treatment helps to you to harmonize and center yourself, so that you can relax and bring yourself back to the here and now.

Settling in, calming down

The adrenal glands are responsible for producing the stress hormone adrenaline. This is a good thing when we really do need the energy and strength to fight or take flight. But since most of us are no longer living in caves among wild animals, it is not always as good a reaction as it once was.

It is not uncommon to face situations that get your adrenaline pumping during the average working day. It could be a minor event, such as temporarily losing an important paper and then finding it. Or it could be an event that rattles you to your very bones – for example, being on the receiving end of a verbal assault by an unhappy customer with a short fuse.

Some of us are in particularly stressful jobs, day after day. But even if you are the "racehorse" type and thoroughly enjoy the energy and buzz, you still need to take care of yourself. Even the best racehorses need time out to rest and relax, and if you don't give this to yourself, who will?

If, in contrast, you prefer peace and quiet rather than energy and buzz, and have a more delicate temperament, you may easily become thrown off-center by events that most others seem to take easily in their stride. Don't condemn yourself, and don't make the "self-improvement" mistake of trying to fit yourself into a mould that does not suit you. That will only add to the stress that you feel and hinder your ability to flower into the unique and valuable being that you are meant to be.

Anytime you are under stress, for any reason, place your hands over the kidneys (see opposite). There is no possibility of overdoing it, so you can return to the treatment often in the day if you like. When you treat yourself in this position with Reiki, you relax and relieve pressure on the adrenal glands, slowing the production of adrenaline. Combining this position with the others shown on the following pages will further support you in developing a clear, positive attitude to yourself and to life.

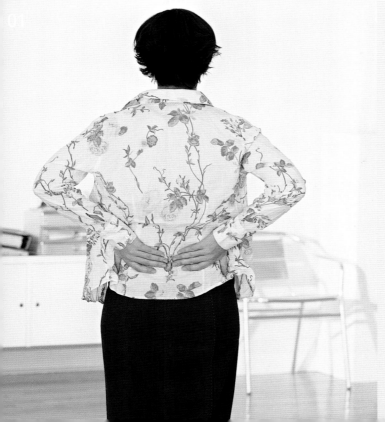

FOR PEACE OF MIND

(01) Place your hands over the kidney area at the back of the waist, fingers relaxed and pointing toward the spine. This position strengthens the kidneys, adrenal glands, and the nerves, as well as relieving stress. It also reinforces self-esteem and confidence.

(02) Place your hands over your eyes, resting your palms on the cheekbones. This helps reduce stress and enhances clarity of thought and intuition.

(03) Place your hands on both sides of your head, above your ears, touching the temples. This harmonizes the two sides of your brain, helps memory, and improves your enjoyment of life.

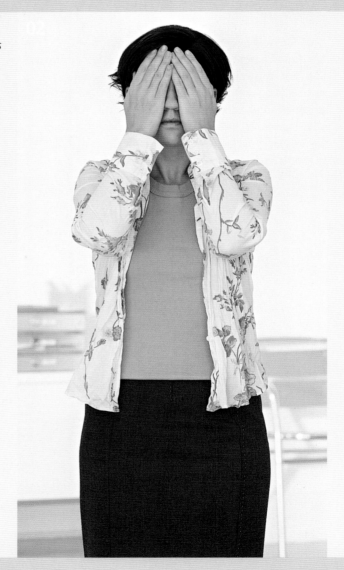

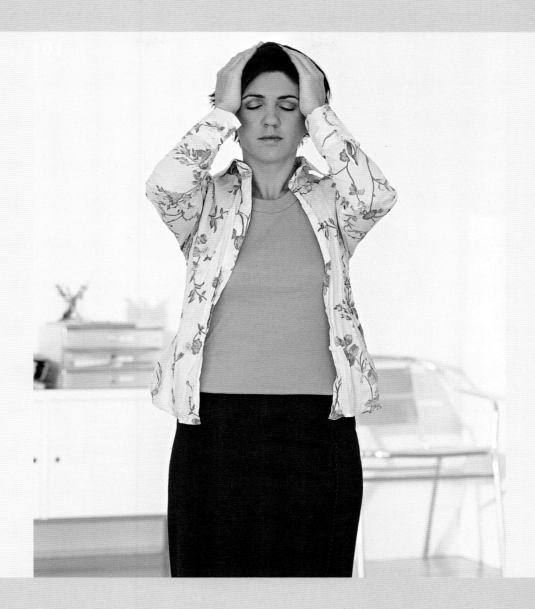

Four quick pick-me-ups

Here, four simple and quick self-treatments have been
selected that you can easily use during the course of
your working day to give yourself a bit of a boost. As
you familiarize yourself with more Reiki treatments, you
will undoubtedly find others that will also help you
with your special needs throughout the day. None of
the treatments draws attention to itself.

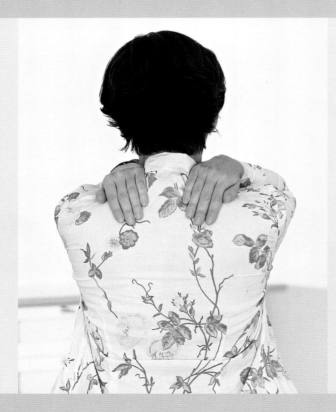

SHOULDER SOOTHER
*If you sit down all day long
at work, you will probably
be all too familiar with the
shoulder tensions, neck, and
back pain that often
accompany sedentary-type
working patterns. Ease that
tension by placing your
hands on the upper
shoulders at either side of
the spine and resting them
there for about 3 minutes,
allowing the Reiki energy to
flow into the places where it
is most needed. This also
helps release any emotions
you might be holding there,
and promotes relaxation.*

BEYOND LUNCH

If you, like many other people, suffer from a noticeable dip in your energy levels after you have eaten lunch, this treatment will help to restore your energy and vitality and get you back on track once more. It has the added benefit of soothing the stomach and digestive system, in the case you have not eaten as wisely as you know you should! Simply lay one hand above, and the other below, the navel. Allow your hands to rest in place for about 3 minutes.

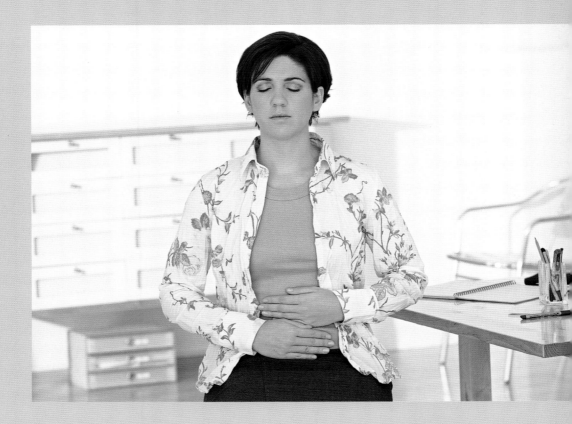

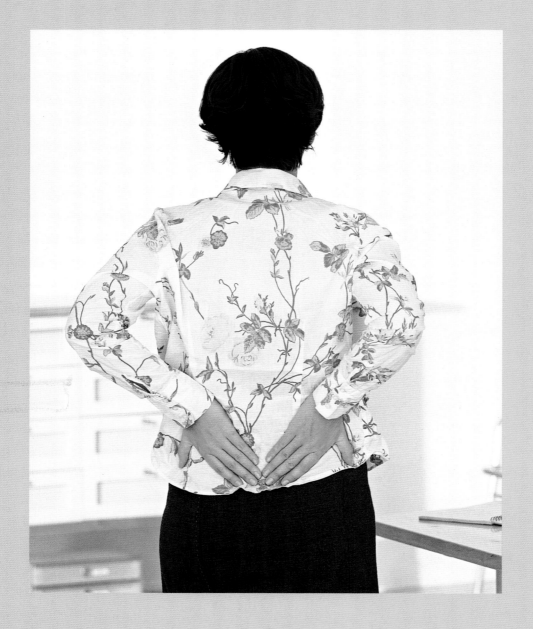

CREATIVITY ENHANCER

If you are feeling stuck while working on a creative problem, or find yourself a bit at sea and not sure about what to do next, try this treatment (see facing page). Place both hands on your back so that your fingers touch the coccyx, with your hands opening into a "V." This treatment promotes creativity and confidence, and supports grounding. It also helps to relieve the effects of sciatic pain.

ENERGY BOOSTER

Frustration, and the tension that comes with it, can make us feel tired and fractious. When it seems that Murphy's Law is operating everywhere you turn, this simple treatment (see right) will help you let go of that frustration and give you the energy you need to start afresh. It also helps digestion, in case the tension has spread to your stomach. Place your hands over the lower part of your ribcage, above the waist. Let them rest in place for a few moments, until you can feel the energy begin to balance and harmonize.

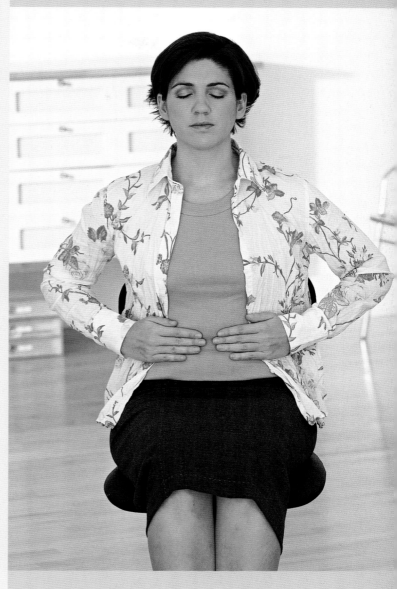

Reiki for colds or flu

When you are suffering from the effects of a cold or flu, or you are feeling hammered by the pain of a headache, it is often a sign that you are overburdened and need to take some time off in order to rest and refresh yourself. Sometimes, however, the pressures on you to perform are such that you simply have to show up at work, even though you may be feeling far from your best.

Here is a simple treatment that you can use to banish your cold or flu symptoms. You can follow this sequence either sitting comfortably in a chair or lying down. You could do this at work, if it were necessary, but it really is best done at home, where you can devote your full attention to the treatment without distractions or interruptions.

The treatment takes about 30 minutes in total and should be done at the beginning and end of your day. During the day you can repeat the head treatments for specific symptoms, as time and space allow.

Headaches are also eased by these hand positions, so make sure you include your shoulders in the treatment (see page 86) if your headache is located primarily at the back of the head.

As you become more sensitive to the signals your body is sending you, you can begin to "catch" these ailments at the very beginning and very often prevent them from developing.

CLEARING YOUR HEAD

Begin treating your head by using head positions in steps 1 to 4. These will ease the inflammation in your sinuses and inner ears, as well as give you general relief for that "stuffy" feeling in the head that accompanies a cold. Stay in each position for about 4 minutes, lengthening to 10 minutes for step 6.

(01) Place your hands over your eyes, resting the palms of your hands on your cheekbones.

(02) Place your hands on both sides of your head, with the palms resting above your ears and touching your temples.

(03) Place your hands on both sides of your head, covering your ears.

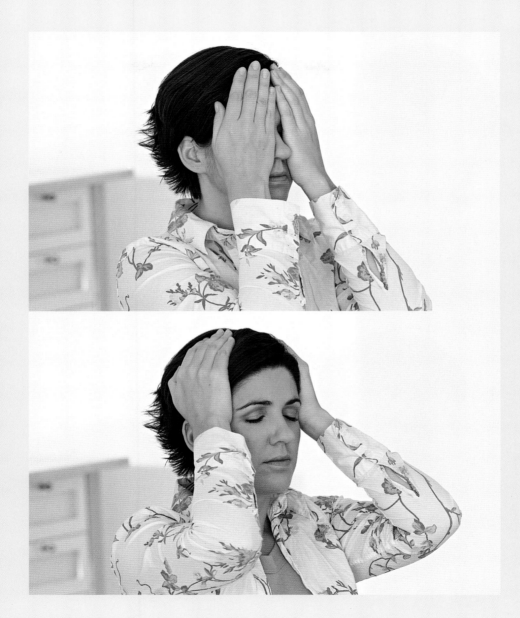

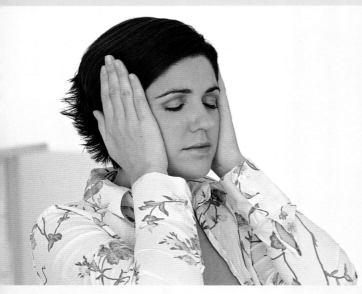

(04) Cup the back of your head in both your hands.

(05) Now lay your hands on either side of your throat. This treats the lymph nodes, helping your body to process and release toxins. It also helps to ease a sore throat.

(06) Place both your hands on the front of your body, below the collarbone, with your fingertips meeting in the middle on the upper part of your breastbone. This position stimulates the thymus gland, which strengthens the immune and lymphatic systems. Let your hands rest in this position for about 10 minutes.

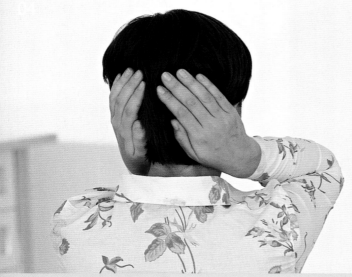

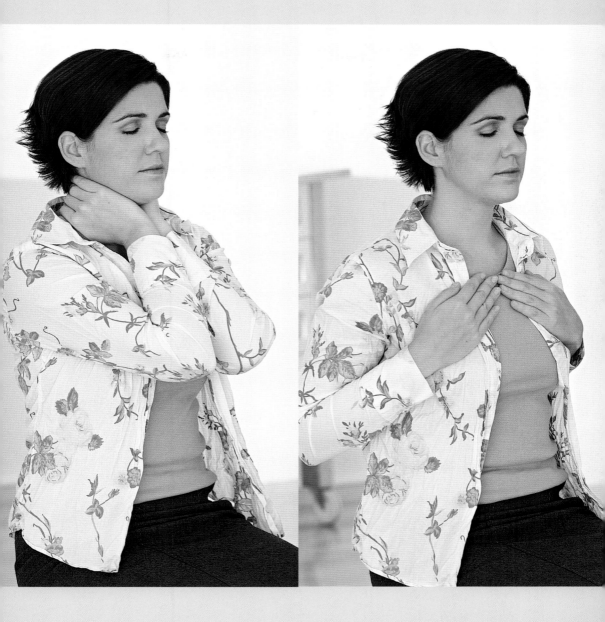

CHAPTER FIVE

Reiki for winding down

Too often at the end of a busy day or a hectic period at work we find it difficult to unwind and relax. So instead of being able to leave work behind we might find ourselves bringing it home – if not in reality, then in our minds.

We cannot seem to stop replaying a meeting that did not go as well as we had hoped, or set aside our concerns about some task we could not manage to complete. Or we arrive home feeling so tired that we find ourselves dreading the night out with friends we had been looking forward to for ages. More often than most of us care to admit, a stressful day leads us straight to the couch, where we escape into mindless television rather than picking up that book we wanted to read.

Making time and space to relax the body, mind, and emotions is essential to staying healthy and avoiding stress-related illnesses and discomforts; it also enhances our overall quality of life and sense of well-being. Even if you are the type of person who thrives on the fast pace of a busy schedule packed with work and social activities, you still need to take time to smell the roses, whatever that might mean for you. We all know, or have heard a story about, a person who was vital, energetic, always on the move, and was never sick – and then suddenly suffered a heart attack. With a little more awareness and attention directed toward using the gaps between your activities to nourish the complexity that you are, this sort of unexpected crisis is much less likely to occur.

The treatments and exercises on the following pages can help you to relax and restore yourself at the end of the day, so that you can devote your evenings and weekends to rewarding yourself for your workday efforts.

Reiki to refresh your energy

This treatment is especially helpful in "changing gears" at the end of the workday, letting go of the day's events, and restoring your energy. If you have a social event on your calendar, or you simply want to spend time enjoying a favorite activity or hobby, giving yourself Reiki healing is a great way to recharge your batteries. This treatment takes about 30 minutes at the most. If you treat yourself on a daily basis, the effect may be even more noticeable. It can also be done sitting in a chair if that is more convenient.

LETTING GO
(01) Lie down and make yourself comfortable. With each exhale, feel your body sinking deeper and deeper into the floor or mattress beneath you.

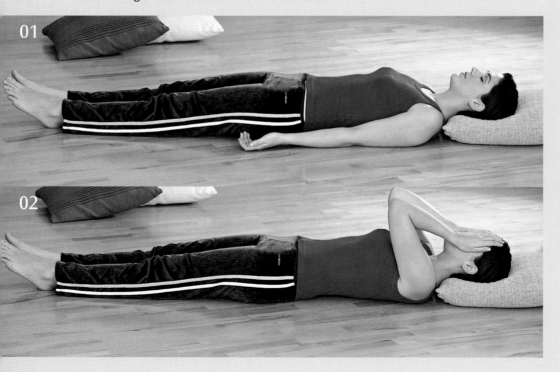

01

02

(02) Lay your hands over your eyes, with your palms resting on your cheekbones. This balances the pituitary and pineal glands, which regulate the hormones that keep us in balance and which support and promote relaxation.

(03) Now place your hands on both sides of your head above your ears, touching the temples with your fingers meeting at or as near as possible the top of your head. This

position eases stress, calms the racing thoughts in your brain, and soothes the mind. It also helps to alleviate the pain and distress of headaches.

(04) Cup the back of your head with both of your hands. This position enhances your sense of security and eases any fears or depression you might be experiencing. It also helps to calm and harmonize the mind and emotions.

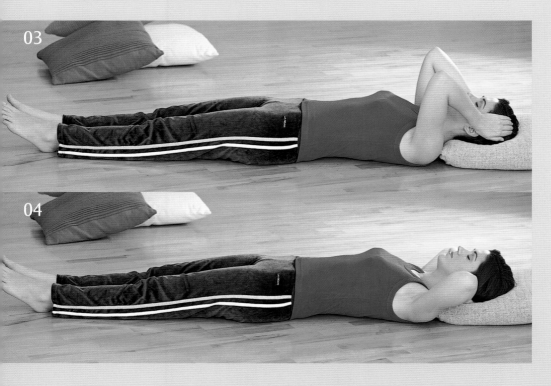

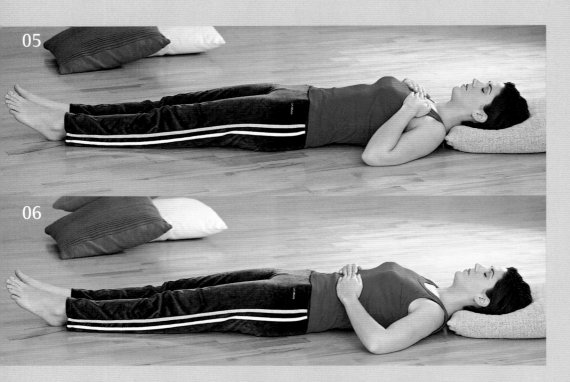

(05) Lay your hands on the left and right sides of your upper chest, fingers touching just below the collarbone. This strengthens the immune system, regulates heart and blood pressure, and stimulates the lymph circulation, which helps to keep the body free of toxins. It also helps to relieve and dissolve negative emotions.

(06) Lay your hands on your solar plexus, over the lower ribcage and above the waist. This position restores energy, promotes relaxation, and reduces feelings of fear and frustration.

(07) Sitting up, place your hands around the waist at the level of your kidneys, with your fingers pointing toward the spine. This position strengthens the kidneys, adrenal glands, and nervous system. It also helps to detoxify the body and promotes relaxation, reinforcing self-esteem and confidence.

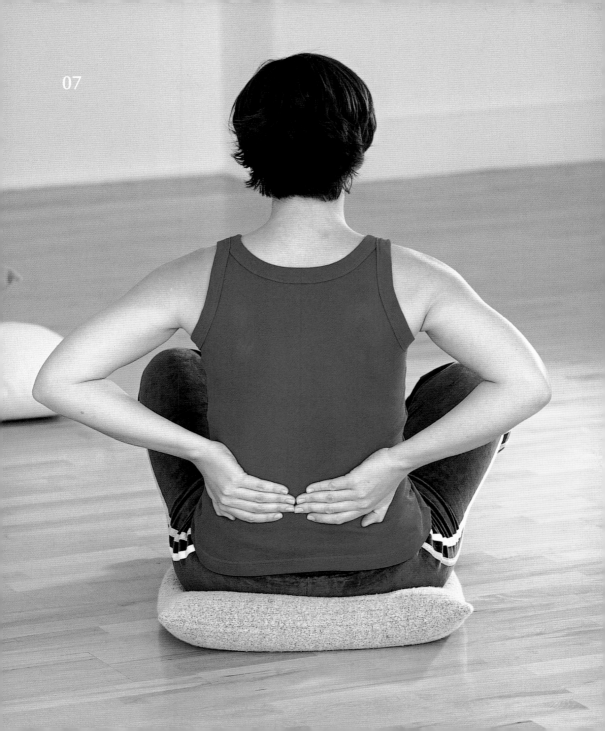

Self-relaxation exercise

Just as a bicycle keeps going for some while even after you have stopped pedalling, you often find yourself still racing even when you are allowed to relax and take a break. Tensions in the body and worries in the mind can prevent you from relaxing and enjoying a good night's rest. This treatment, which combines Reiki and a visualization exercise, helps to relax tensions in the body and the mind. It can be done before you go to sleep, or at any time during the day, over a few days, if you feel that lately your wheels have been spinning too fast.

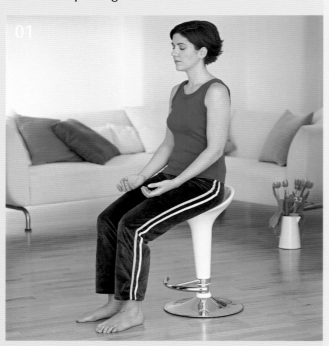

RELAX AND UNWIND

(01) Sit comfortably in a chair with your feet flat on the floor, or lie down. Take a few deep breaths, breathing in through your nose and out through your mouth. Allow yourself to make a little sigh with each exhale. Feel your whole body relaxing and letting go of tension.

(02) Now place your hands over your eyes, with your palms resting on your cheekbones. After about 3 minutes, keeping your hands over your eyes, turn your awareness to your feet. Begin to visualize and watch, with your eyes still closed, the energy coming up through your feet. Watch from inside to see if there is any tension in your feet and, if you find it, consciously let it go and relax your feet. Don't move on from this point until you feel that relaxation has really come.

(03) Now move your attention, in turn, to your ankles, calves, knees, thighs, and hips, and see if there is any tension in any of these areas. Again, consciously relax and let go of any tensions that you find there.

In the same way, move slowly up through all the different parts of your body – the groin, belly, buttocks, all the organs, lungs, shoulders, arms – and as each part relaxes, feel the energy flowing into and through you.

Notice what is happening in your hands – your hands are connected to your brain. Tensions in the right hand reflect tensions in the left side of the brain, and tensions in the left hand mirror tensions in the right side of the brain. Relax your face, the skin of your head, your neck. Finally, look to see if there are any tensions in the mind. You will find that just by watching, the tensions and thoughts begin to disappear. When your whole body is relaxed, your mind is relaxed, too.

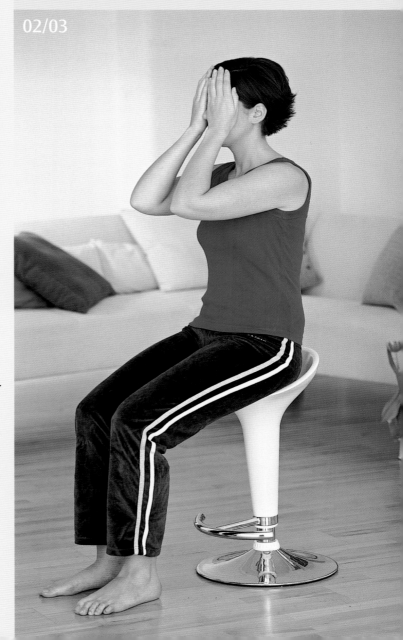

02/03

Healing relaxation

This exercise can help you guide yourself into a
healing relaxation. Be sure to create a private space
for yourself so that you will not be disturbed – turn
off the phone, close the door, and make it known to
anyone who shares your living space that you should
not be interrupted for about half an hour. This
exercise is particularly good for times when you feel
depleted and out of balance, and you're not quite sure
what the cause is or what to do to bring yourself back
to a healthy place.

   You can play soothing music throughout – Gregorian
chants are good, as is overtone singing or mantra
singing. For vocal music, it is best that the words do
not carry content that takes the attention of your
mind away from the exercise itself. If this music does
not appeal, then you can choose any type of
instrumental music that feels particularly healing to
you. You can also record the relevant parts of the
instructions in your own voice, leaving gaps of silence
between the different steps.

**ENTERING A HEALING
STATE**
*(01) Lie down comfortably
and relax, with your eyes
closed. Cover yourself with a
blanket or sheet. Otherwise,
as you relax more deeply and
your metabolism slows
down, you might start to feel
chilled. Take a few deep
breaths and let go of any
thoughts or tensions in the
body each time you breathe
out. Feel your body sinking
deeper into the floor with
each exhale.*

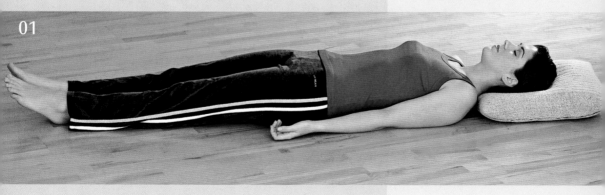

01

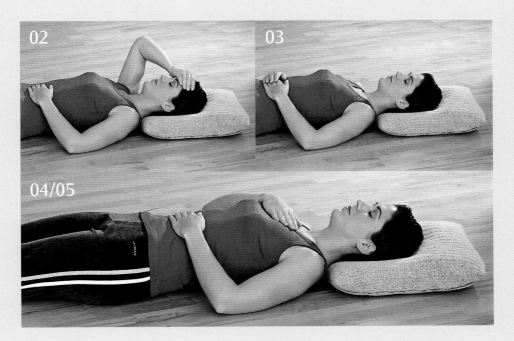

(02) Place your hands anywhere on your body where it feels right, or where you feel that you need some support. Allow Reiki energy to flow into your body. Now sink inside yourself and allow yourself to relax even more deeply. Remain for 2 to 3 minutes in this state.

(03) Slowly move your hands to another part of your body and allow Reiki energy to flow into you there. Remain like this for another 2 to 3 minutes.

(04) Move your attention to the inside of your body and explore it. If you come across any dark corners, notice them. Simply notice them, without putting a label on them or

making any type of judgment. Now send some light to these dark areas. Let the light enter from the top of your head (the crown chakra) and allow it to flow into your body. Also let the light emanate from your hands into your body.

(05) Now sink even more deeply inside yourself. Let yourself be touched by something higher than you, higher than your personality, a divine force, a divine energy. Going even deeper into an unknown space inside yourself, the healing that is needed for you can happen now. Allow another 10 minutes, with or without music, for the relaxation and healing to take place.

Prayer Meditation

This particular meditation is best done at night, in a darkened room, to be followed immediately by a period of restful, restorative sleep. If you would rather do it in the morning, then you should allow for about 15 minutes' rest afterward.

The exercise is called the Prayer Meditation because it connects you very directly and deeply to the powerful healing energy of the universe.

RESTORATIVE MEDITATION

(01) Kneel down and raise both your hands, with your palms face up and your head raised. Feel cosmic energy flowing into you; fill yourself with the energy of the sky. Be like a leaf in the breeze, allowing yourself to tremble, if it happens, as the energy flows down your arms. Let your whole body vibrate with this energy.

(02) When you are completely filled, usually after 2 or 3 minutes, bend down and let your forehead touch the ground, with your arms stretched out in front of you and your palms face down on the floor. Become a vehicle, allowing the energy of the sky to unite with the energy of the earth.

Repeat the first and second steps at least 7 times, more if possible. It is important to repeat the steps at least 7 times because otherwise you are likely to feel restless and unable to sleep.

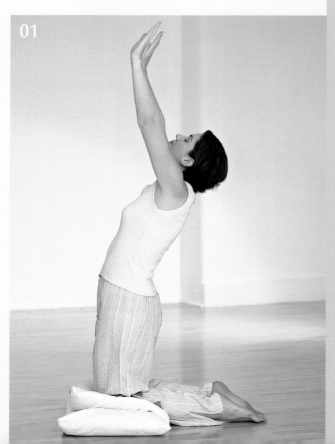

01

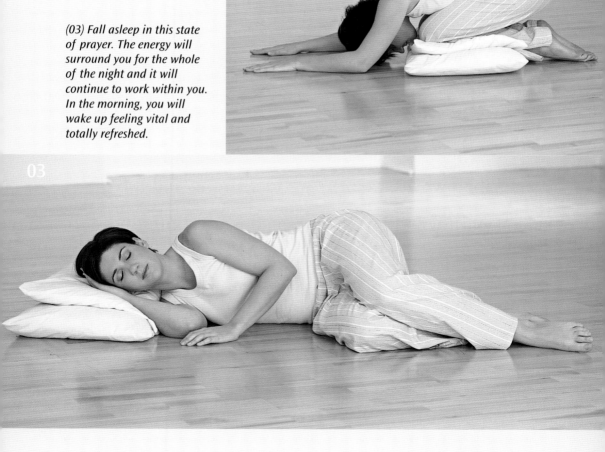

(03) Fall asleep in this state of prayer. The energy will surround you for the whole of the night and it will continue to work within you. In the morning, you will wake up feeling vital and totally refreshed.

CHAPTER SIX

Reiki healing hands

When we are healthy we feel strong and full of vitality and joy. We are balanced, contented, and in harmony with ourselves. When we fall out of tune, our bodies can respond by creating a symptom or illness.

Disturbances that cause us to fall out of tune most often start in the mind, and are later mirrored in the body. Thus, in order to understand the phenomenon of health and illness, we must think of a person as a whole, made up of body, mind, emotions, and soul. The body is the earthly material part, the physical house for the soul. The mind, emotions, and soul, or spirit, are the subtle aspects.

Every illness has a specific message for us. The first thing we must do is recognize and accept that message. It is most important not to reject or repress the illness, but to understand its signals. If we can accept the challenge and are honest with ourselves, we can learn from the experience. We have taken the first step toward healing.

The gift of Reiki is that it supports healing on all levels. Before a problem in the body shows itself as an illness, it announces itself in the psyche as a theme, idea, wish, or fantasy. The next time you get a cold, take note of what has been going on in your psyche – perhaps you were feeling overwhelmed at work, and wished you could take a few days off. Or maybe, out of a sense of obligation or duty, you accepted an invitation to a social event and then immediately regret having done so. The cold could be the body's way of cooperating with your wish.

By respecting and loving our bodies, and by tending to our emotional and spiritual needs, we experience healing. Sensing what we need to feel content, fit, and healthy brings us closer to ourselves and strengthens our will to live.

Self-treatments

You can use Reiki self-treatment simply and effectively on yourself at all times. The techniques opposite and on the following pages show the entire self-treatment sequence, and it can be done either sitting comfortably in a chair or lying down. The entire sequence takes between 45 and 60 minutes to complete. Remain in each position for about 3 to 5 minutes – allow your instincts to determine the precise timing. Keep your hands slightly cupped and relaxed, so that they can follow the curves of your body, with the fingers closed. Start with the head, working down the front of the body, and end by treating the back.

If you have pain or special problem areas, allow your hands to rest longer on these spots – say, between 10 and 20 minutes. And if an area of the body feels particularly warm or cold, this may be a sign of imbalance. You can allow your hands to rest longer in that spot until you feel that the energy is becoming more harmonious once more. Allow your intuition to be your guide.

As you experiment with these treatments and learn how your body, mind, and emotions respond to them, you can also use them individually, or in combination, to treat specific symptoms or discomforts.

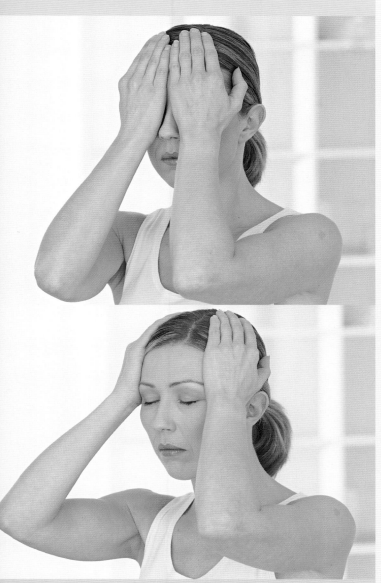

TREATING YOUR HEAD
Head Position One
Place your hands over your eyes, resting your palms on your cheekbones. This position helps colds, supports intuition and clarity of thought, and reduces stress. It also supports meditation, and can be done as an isolated position before you meditate.

Head Position Two
Place your hands on both sides of your head above your ears, touching your temples with the heels of the hands. This position harmonizes the two sides of the brain, improves memory and enjoyment of life, and is helpful for depression and the pain of headaches.

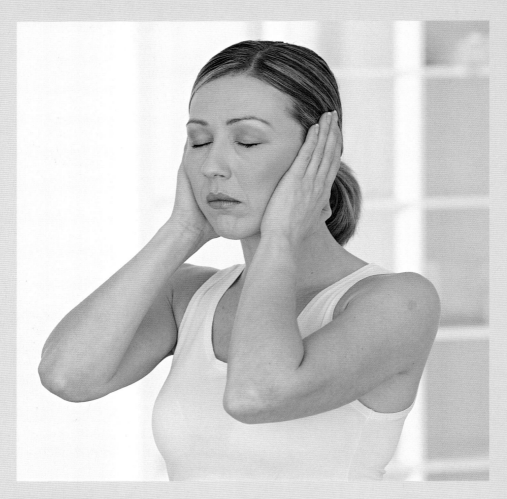

Head Position Three
Place your hands on both sides of your head, covering your ears. This position promotes a deep sense of comfort and relaxes the whole body. It is also helpful for earache and easing the symptoms of colds and flu.

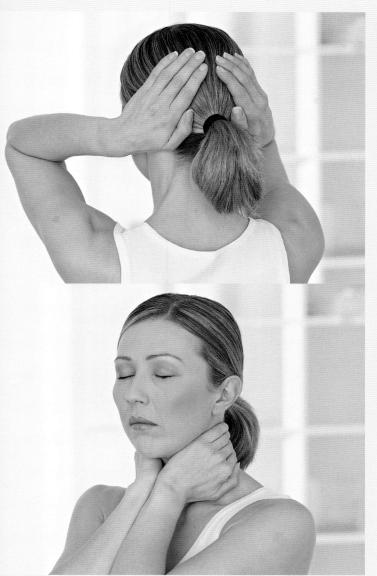

Head Position Four

Place both your hands on the back of your head, as if you are holding a ball. This position helps to ease sleep disorders and supports a feeling of security and freedom from fears. It also supports intuition, relieves depression, and calms the mind and emotions.

Head Position Five

Place your hands on both sides of your neck, with your wrists touching each other at the middle of your throat. This position harmonizes blood pressure and metabolism, helps ease neck pains and hoarseness, and promotes self-expression.

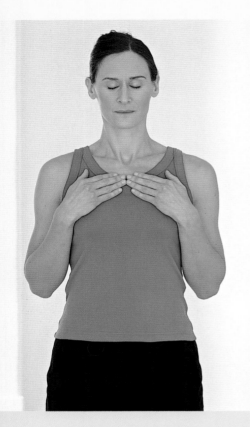

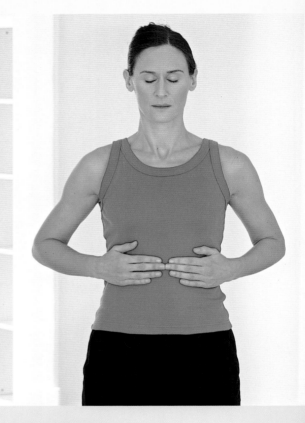

TREATING YOUR FRONT
Front Position One
Place your hands on the left and right sides of your upper chest, fingers touching just below the collarbone. This position strengthens the immune system, regulates heart and blood pressure, stimulates lymph circulation, and transforms negativity, increasing your capacity for love and the enjoyment of life.

Front Position Two
Place both your hands over your lower ribcage, above the waist, with your fingers touching. This position helps to regulate the digestion, refreshes and revitalizes energy, promotes relaxation, and reduces fears and frustrations.

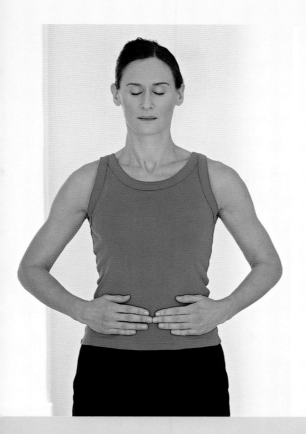

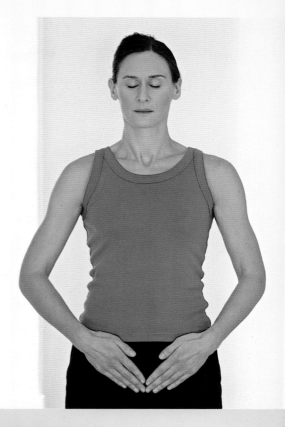

Front Position Three

Place your hands at the navel, with your fingers touching. This position regulates digestion, sugar and fat metabolism (pancreas), and helps to ease powerful emotions, such as fears, depressions, and frustrations. It also helps to increase self-confidence.

Front Position Four

Place your hands over the pubic bone, in the shape of a "V" – for women, the fingers should touch. For men, your hands should rest on the top of each thigh. This position treats the large intestine, bladder, urethra, and sexual organs. It eases menstrual disorders in women, provides grounding, and helps to ease existential fear.

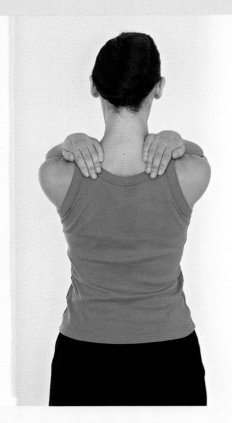

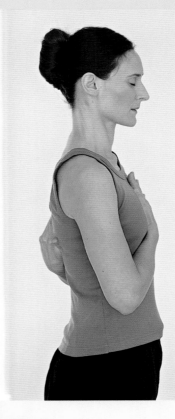

TREATING YOUR BACK
Back Position One
Place your hands on your upper shoulders, at either side of your spine. This position is helpful in easing shoulder tension and back and neck problems. It promotes relaxation, releases blocked emotions, and helps difficulties that are to do with "shouldering" responsibility.

Back Position Two
Place one hand with your palm resting on the center of your chest, over the middle of the heart, and the other at the same height on your back. This position balances and harmonizes the thymus gland and the heart, stimulates the immune system, and increases confidence and the enjoyment of life. It also helps to alleviate worries and depression.

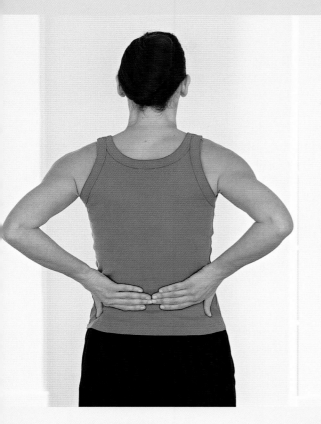

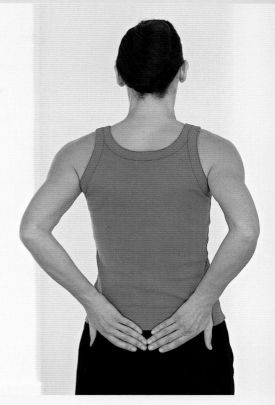

Back Position Three
Place your hands around your waist at the height of your kidneys, with your fingers pointing toward the spine. This strengthens the kidneys, adrenal glands, and nerves, and helps to cleanse the body of toxins. It also relieves stress, eases back pains, and reinforces self-esteem and confidence.

Back Position Four
Place the heels of your hands at the back of your waist, with the fingers pointing down in a "V" shape so that the tips of the fingers touch your coccyx. This position treats the sexual organs, helps digestion, and eases discomfort in the sciatic nerve. It also promotes creativity and confidence, and helps grounding.

Treating others

Reiki is a powerful healing art that supports and brings harmony to individuals so that they can share a deep love and understanding with others. To give and receive love is an important human need. When we are able to express love toward ourselves and others, it literally supports health and well-being. But just as we need to love ourselves first before we can truly love others, we need to be healthy ourselves before we can truly serve as a channel for the universal life energy in giving Reiki treatments to others.

This is one of the reasons why the energy attunement given by a Reiki Master-Teacher is so important. Even if you have not yet received training and initiation in Reiki, you can still share Reiki treatments with your friends and loved ones. The treatments will, however, be most beneficial if you first deepen your own awareness of the effects of Reiki by treating yourself over a period of time (see pages 108–15). In this way, you develop the first-hand experience, sensitivity, and intuitive understanding of the subtle energies that are required to support relaxation and healing in yourself as well as in others.

PREPARING FOR AND GIVING A REIKI TREATMENT

When treating another person, remain in each hand position for between 3 and 5 minutes. In time and with the benefit of the experience it brings, you will be able to sense exactly when a particular part of the body has received sufficient Reiki treatment. If your partner has specific problem areas or symptoms, you can treat those areas for about 10 or 20 minutes.

PREPARATIONS FOR A REIKI TREATMENT

- *Clean and prepare the room.*
- *Have a blanket ready in case of cold.*
- *If you are the giver or receiver, take off your watch and any jewelry.*
- *Make sure that all phones are switched off.*
- *If you are the receiver, remove your shoes and loosen tight clothing. If wearing a belt, remove it.*
- *Relax and center yourself before starting the treatment.*
- *Rinse your hands in cold running water before and after a treatment.*
- *Play relaxing music, or opt for silence instead.*
- *If you are the receiver, keep your legs uncrossed.*
- *If you are the giver, remind yourself before and afterwards that you are being used as a channel for healing energy.*
- *Afterwards, smooth the aura 3 times and draw an energy line from the coccyx up over the head. Allow the receiver to rest for a while.*

Again, your intuition will tell you when it is time to move on to the next area to treat. When your hands are in a problem area, you might feel a sensation of heat or cold. In that case, let your hands rest in place until you sense that the energy flow has normalized.

Your hands are laid gently and lightly on your partner, with your fingers together. A complete treatment covering the head, front, back, and legs will take between an hour and an hour and a half. The Reiki short treatment, shown on pages 129–34, takes about half an hour to complete.

AURA SMOOTHING
At the beginning of a Reiki treatment, stroke the receiver's aura in a smooth, curving form, starting at the head and working down to the feet. This has a relaxing effect on the receiver and prepares him or her for the treatment to follow.

TREATING THE HEAD

A full Reiki treatment usually starts with treating the head. The head positions have a particularly strong effect, relaxing and balancing the entire body. In addition to their use in a full Reiki treatment, the individual head positions can also be used alone or in combination to ease the specific symptoms and discomforts that are described.

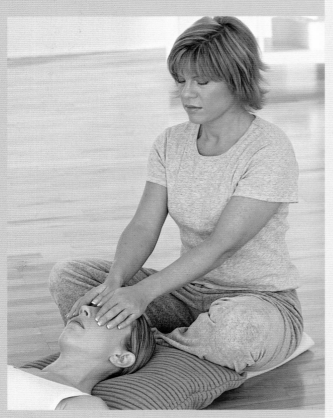

Head Position One

Lay your hands to the right and left of the nose, covering the forehead, eyes, and cheeks. This position balances the pituitary and pineal glands, and is good for treating the eyes and sinuses. It can be used to treat exhaustion, stress, colds, sinus disorders, eye disorders, and allergies. Relaxing the eyes helps to ease the whole body. If your receiver wishes, you can lay a tissue over the forehead, extending down to either side of the nostrils, before giving the treatment.

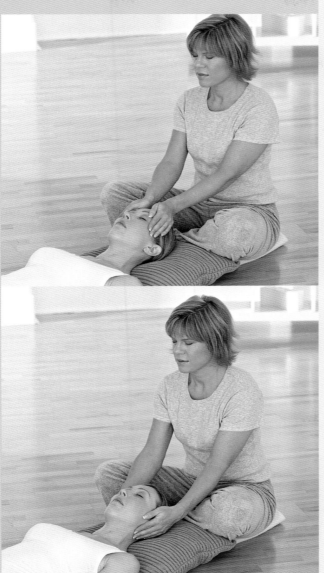

Head Position Two

Lay your hands over the temples, with your palms following the shape of the head, so that your fingertips touch the outside edges of the cheekbones. This position balances the right and left sides of the brain and body, and is good for treating the eye muscles and nerves. It helps to ease stress, slows down racing or confused thoughts and worries, and helps learning and concentration. It also helps to alleviate the symptoms of colds and headaches.

Head Position Three

Place your hands so that the centers of your palms are over the ears. This position is good for treating the pharynx and disturbances to the sense of balance. It also helps disorders of the outer and inner ear, eases symptoms such as noise or hissing in the ears, poor hearing, disorders of the nose and throat, and colds and flu.

Head Position Four

Hold the back of the head with your fingertips over the medulla oblongata, where the spine meets the back of the skull. This position is good for treating tensions in the back of the head and irritations of the eyes and nose. It helps calm powerful emotions, such as fear and shock, and promotes calm and clear thinking. Use it to relieve tension headaches, eye disorders, colds, asthma, hay fever, and digestive disorders.

Head Position Five

Lay your hands at the sides and above the front part of the throat, but do not touch it directly. This position is good for treating the thyroid and parathyroid glands, larynx, vocal cords, and lymph nodes. It is used to treat metabolic disorders, weight problems, heart palpitations and fibrillation, high or low blood pressure, sore throat, inflamed tonsils, flu, and hoarseness. It also helps self-expression and balances repressed or uncontrolled feelings of aggression.

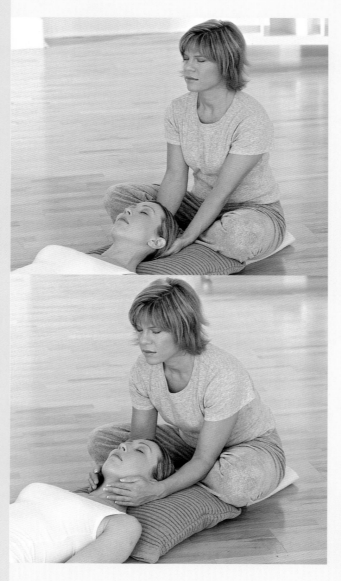

TREATING THE FRONT OF THE BODY

Working on this area of the body deepens the whole healing process in a full Reiki treatment. Emotional reactions may happen during this part of the treatment, though they are not inevitable. The front positions help to balance the organs and stimulate the chakras. As with the head positions, the front positions can be used individually or in combination to ease the specific symptoms described.

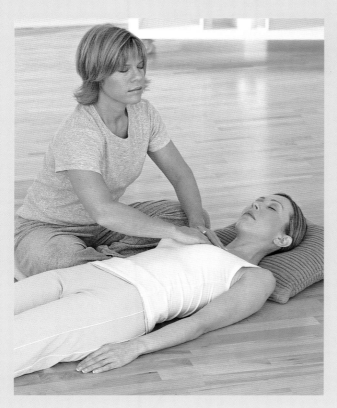

Front Position One

Lay one hand across the thymus gland below the collarbone. Lay the other hand at a right angle to the first on the breastbone, in the middle of the chest, forming a "T" shape. This position is good for treating the thymus gland, heart, and lungs, and fortifies the immune and lymph systems. It is also good for bronchitis, deafness, general weakness, and depression.

Front Position Two

Lay one hand on the lower ribs on the right side, and the other hand just below this hand at the waist. This position treats the liver and gall bladder, pancreas, duodenum, and parts of the stomach and large intestine. It helps to ease symptoms, including those of hepatitis, gall stones, digestive and metabolic disorders, and aids detoxification of the body. It also balances emotions, such as anger and depression.

Front Position Three

Lay one hand on the lower ribs on the left side, and the other hand just below this hand at the waist. This position is good for treating the spleen, parts of the pancreas, large intestine, small intestine, and stomach. It is used for disorders of the pancreas or spleen and for diabetes, flu, infections, digestive problems, anaemia, and leukaemia. It also helps to stabilize the immune system.

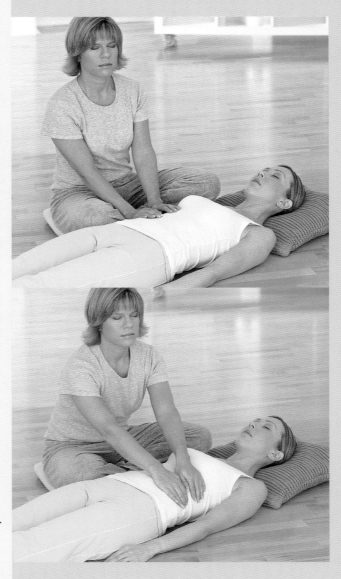

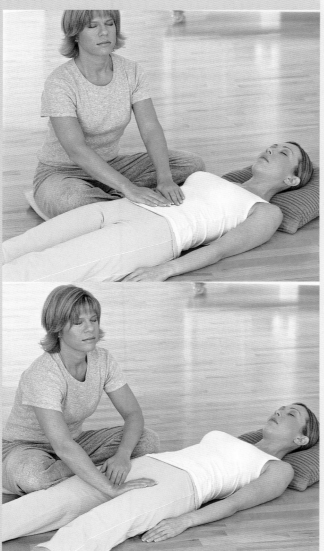

Front Position Four

Lay one hand above and the other below the navel. This position is used to treat the solar plexus, stomach, digestive system, lymphatic system, and intestines. It helps to relieve intestinal disorders, nausea, indigestion, bloated feelings, and metabolic disorders. It is also good for restoring energy and vitality, and helps to ease powerful emotions, such as depression, fear, and shock.

Front Position Five

For men, place your hands in the groin area, without touching the penis. For women, lay both hands over the pubic bone. This position is used for treating the abdominal organs, intestines, bladder, and urethra. It eases urogenital, menstrual, and menopausal disorders, appendix and digestive disorders, cramps, back pain, and problems with the uterus, bladder, and prostate gland.

TREATING THE BACK OF THE BODY

Having this part of your body treated helps you to let go of tensions, thoughts, and feelings. When the receiver is lying face down, they tend to feel more protected and secure, so healing and relaxation can take place at deeper levels. All positions can also be used individually and in combination to treat the particular symptoms described.

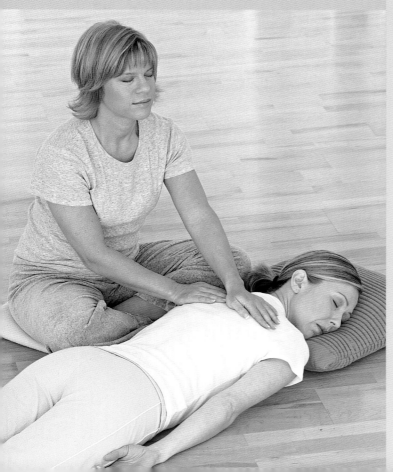

Back Position One

(Unillustrated) Lay both hands on the shoulders, one hand to the left and the other to the right of the spine. This position is good for treating tensions and discomfort in the neck and the shoulder muscles. It is also helpful in easing stress, difficulties with responsibility, and bringing blocked emotions into consciousness, where they can be dealt with.

Back Position Two

Lay your hands on the shoulder blades. This position is good for treating the shoulders, heart, lungs, and the upper back. It is used for coughs and bronchitis, as well as back and shoulder pain. It also helps to sooth powerful emotional upsets and promotes the capacity for love, confidence, and enjoyment.

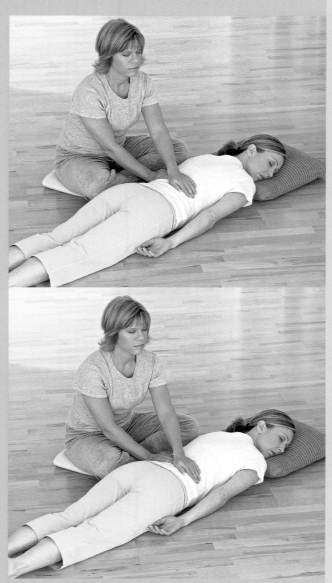

Back Position Three

Lay your hands on the lower ribs above the kidneys. This position treats the adrenal glands, kidneys, and nervous system. It can be used for kidney disorders and allergies, and helps in the detoxification of the body. It is also good for treating the shock from emergencies and accidents, fear, and stress. When tensions held in the lower back are released, we can more easily let go of the past and of stress and pain.

Back Position Four

When the receiver has a long back, you can also lay your hands on the lower part of the back at hip level. This position helps to treat sciatica and lower back pain, in addition to strengthening the nerves and lymph system. It also supports creativity and sexuality, and eases hip problems.

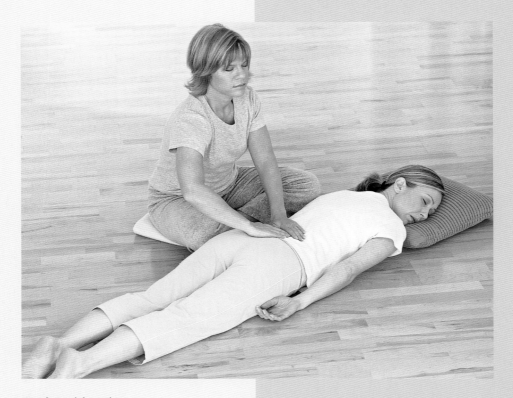

Back Position Five

Lay one hand across the sacrum, the other at right angles to the first, over the coccyx, forming a "T" shape. This position is good for treating the intestines, urogenital system, and sciatic nerve, and is used for hemorrhoids, digestive problems, intestinal inflammations, bladder disorders, prostate problems, vaginal disorders, and sciatic pain. It is also good for easing existential fears.

TREATING THE LEGS

The legs and feet carry the whole weight of the body, and problems with the legs, knees, and feet can be symptomatic of a hesitation and fear of moving forward in life. Emotions are also stored in the upper and lower legs. Treatment of the legs can release blocked energy and bring to the awareness of the receiver what needs to be done to move forward in directions that will be most beneficial and healing.

Knee Hollow Position
Cover the hollows of the knees with your hands. This position is good for treating all parts of the knee joint, easing sports injuries and other types of damage, and unblocking the flow of energy from the feet to the lower back. It also eases fears, especially the fear of dying.

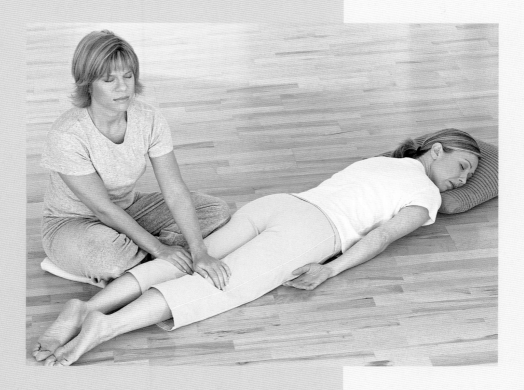

Sole Position A

Lay your hands on the soles of the feet, with the fingertips covering the toes. In reflexology, the soles of the feet are connected with all the organs, and treating them helps grounding and overall vitality.

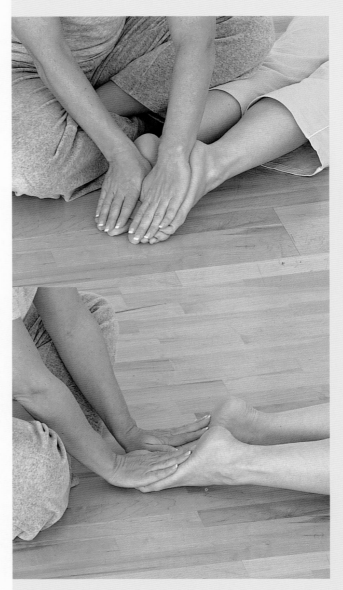

Sole Position B

Rest the heels of your hands on the toes and point your fingertips toward the heels. This position has the same effect as Sole Position A, and will help the receiver to sense a strengthened energy flow from feet to head, as the body is experienced as a whole.

REIKI SHORT TREATMENT

This simple Reiki treatment is good for relieving feelings of stress, easing headaches, and balancing the chakras. It also eases tensions and refreshes energy levels and vitality. The entire treatment will take between 35 and 45 minutes. If you don't have that much free time available, you can end the treatment with Position Seven. This will reduce the total treatment time to about 25 minutes.

Ask the receiver to sit comfortably with their legs uncrossed and their hands resting on the thighs. At the beginning and the end of the treatment, stroke the aura (see pages 18–19 and 117) from the head to the foot. This has a calming and relaxing effect, especially if you take the last stroke from the sacral region up over the top of the head.

Position One
Lay your hands gently on the shoulders, centering yourself and sending love to the receiver.

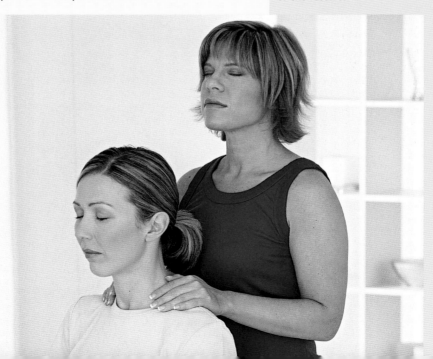

Position Two

*Lay your hands on the cap of
the skull, leaving the crown
(7th chakra) free.*

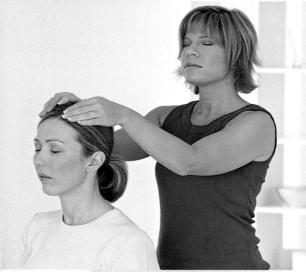

Position Three

*Lay one hand on the back of
the neck, the other hand on
the forehead.*

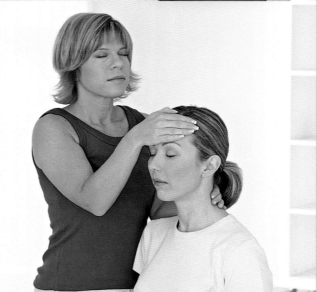

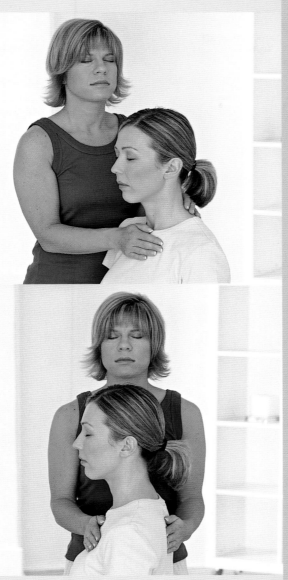

Position Four

*Lay one hand on the 7th
neck vertebra – this is the
vertebra at the base of the
neck and top of the spine
that protrudes outward –
and the other hand at the
front, on the hollow below
the Adam's apple.*

Position Five

*Lay one hand at the center
of the chest over the breast
bone/heart center) and the
other at the same height on
the back, between the
shoulder blades.*

Position Six

Lay one hand on the front of the body, covering the solar plexus, and the other at the same height at the center of the back.

Position Seven

Lay one hand below the navel, and the other hand at the same height over the sacral region.

You can end this short treatment at this position, or, if you still have a few minutes to spare, you can use the remaining positions for a more comprehensive treatment.

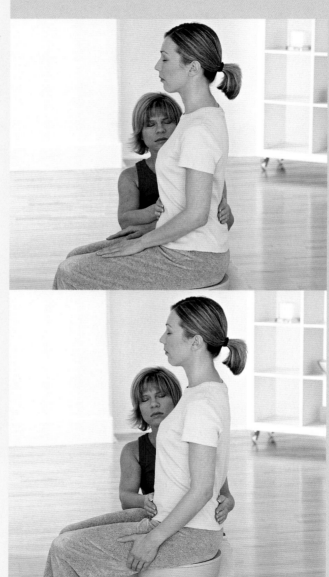

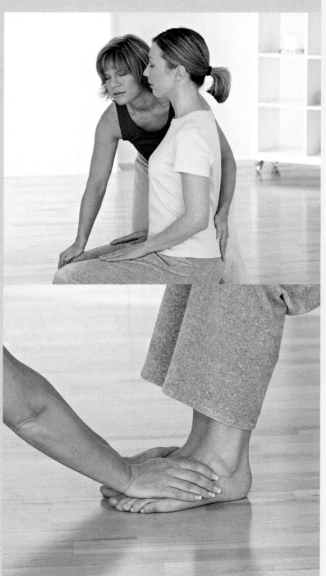

Position Eight

Lay one hand on the sacrum, with your fingertips pointing downward. Place the other hand on one knee. Then change sides and treat the other knee.

Position Nine

Lay your hands on the feet as shown, with your thumbs touching and your fingers encompassing the whole of the instep.

Position Ten

Lay one hand on the upper back between the shoulder blades at the level of the heart center. Lay the other hand at the front over the solar plexus.

Position Eleven

Lay one hand on the middle back, just about at waist height and at the level of the kidneys, and the other at the same height on the front of the stomach.

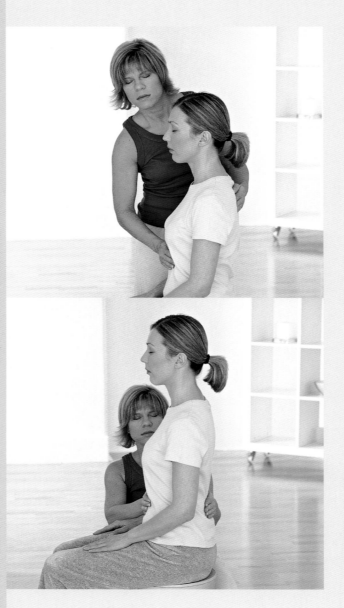

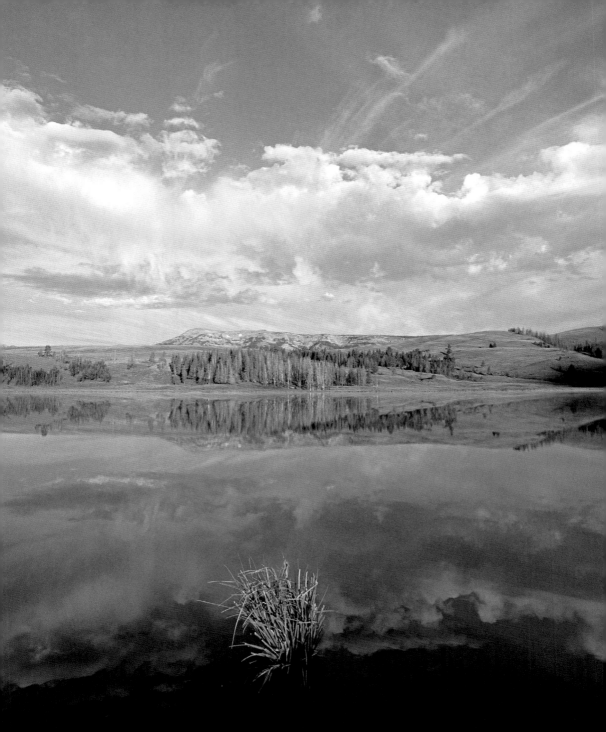

Glossary

Affirmation
Usually a phrase or word describing a positive condition that we wish for ourselves.

Attunements
Special initiations in the Reiki energy, also known as energy transmissions. These open a channel for the healing energies in the chakras.

Aura
The energy field surrounding the body; a subtle, invisible essence. The human aura can be rendered visible by Kirlian photography.

Chakra
Circular energy centers in the human subtle body. There are seven main chakras and they are located in the etheric body. The chakras are known as: root (first); sacral (second); solar plexus (third); heart (fourth); throat (fifth); third eye (sixth); and crown (seventh). The word *chakra* comes from the Sanskrit, meaning "wheel." On the physical plane the chakras coincide approximately with the body's endocrine system.

Channel
A person whose inner healing channel has been opened to the subtle energies of Reiki, so that they can flow through him or her, to be used for self-healing or the healing of others.

Distant healing
Allows you to send healing energies on a mental level over a distance. Similar to radio and television signals, healing energy is sent as though over a "golden bridge."

Enlightened
Describes somebody who has experienced and lives his or her own divinity, and has witnessed inner "light." The presence of an enlightened one is a constant, permanent, selfless state. Also known as a mystic, guru, or saint, such as St. Francis of Assisi, for example.

Etheric body
The energetic counterpart of the physical body, in which the chakras are located.

Forehead chakra
Also known as the third eye; it is responsible for clairvoyance, telepathy, and spiritual awakening. Its activity is stimulated by meditation.

Higher self
The part of every person that is divine. We receive guidance from our

higher self when, for example, we are engaged in mental healing.

Kirlian photography
A special method, developed by S. Kirlian in Russia, allowing the aura to become visible through photography.

Life force energy
The vital energy of life in all living things.

Light energy
Describes the fact that in nature the basic substance of all things is energy, and energy in its essence can be described as "light." In Reiki, this light energy is activated from within.

Mantras
Words and sounds that cause subtle energies to vibrate. These are used in meditations and in Reiki energy transmissions.

Meditation
A state of "not thinking" – "the awakening of the inner witness." Meditation happens in the present and is an immediate state of "not wanting, not doing." It is the ultimate state of relaxation.

Mental healing
Healing through the mind, by the emission of gathered mental energy. Can also take place in the form of distant healing.

Meridian
The name for energy lines running through the entire body that transport life energy to the organs. By stimulating a meridian you balance and activate the function of each organ.

Mystic
See Enlightened.

Om
Holy sound or mantra used in religious ceremonies and meditations.

Reflexology
A massage technique treating parts of the body's organs by massaging the soles of the feet, where the reflex zones of the organs are located.

Sacrum
The bone plate above the cleft of the buttocks.

Sanskrit
Ancient Indian language.

Spiritual healing
The use of cosmic universal energy for treating the person. It differs from Reiki only in that in Reiki, a special attunement process is used to create higher vibrations in the giver.

Subconscious
The parts within us that are unknown to us. Containing repressed energies, memories, themes, belief systems, and fears. The subconscious largely governs our behavior.

Subtle body
The part of the body that is invisible to "normal" sight and is charged with higher vibration – a layered energy field permeating and enveloping the physical body. It is thought to be composed of increasingly refined frequencies. The different bands of frequencies form the subtle bodies, each with different properties, all essential for the development and maintenance of a complete human being.

Sufis
Adherents of various Muslim mystical orders.

Superconscious
A level within us that is conscious, full of light, and corresponds with the higher self, which knows and sees things clearly. Also known as intuition or spiritual guidance.

Sutra
A word from Sanskrit meaning "thread," theorem, or textbook. Sutras are also used in contemplation.

Symbols
A symbol comprises a pictorial drawing and a name, or mantra. The Reiki symbols work on the body's healing channel, setting it to vibrate, so increasing the vibrational frequency of the entire body.

Thymus gland
A gland of the endocrine system, which, when activated, stimulates the human immune system.

Universal life energy
The energy of Reiki. The basic energy composing the whole manifest universe and lying behind everything that we are aware of. When it animates a living organism it becomes the life force.

Vibration frequency
The frequency of the vibration of our vital energy, increased by attunement to Reiki.

Index

Tanmaya welcomes hearing from Reiki students and readers, and she can be contacted via www.school-of-usui-reiki.com or by calling +44 (0) 1769 580899. Or, write to her at:

School of Usui Reiki
PO Box 2
Chulmleigh
Devon
UK EX18 7SS